The Endoscopic Oncologist

Editors

KENNETH J. CHANG
JASON B. SAMARASENA

GASTROINTESTINAL ENDOSCOPY CLINICS OF NORTH AMERICA

www.giendo.theclinics.com

Consulting Editor
CHARLES J. LIGHTDALE

January 2024 • Volume 34 • Number 1

ELSEVIER

1600 John F. Kennedy Boulevard • Suite 1800 • Philadelphia, Pennsylvania, 19103-2899

http://www.theclinics.com

GASTROINTESTINAL ENDOSCOPY CLINICS OF NORTH AMERICA Volume 34, Number 1
January 2024 ISSN 1052-5157, ISBN-13: 9780443184116

Editor: Kerry Holland
Developmental Editor: Isha Singh

Gastrointestinal Endoscopy Clinics of North America (ISSN 1052-5157) is published quarterly by Elsevier Inc., 360 Park Avenue South, New York, NY 10010-1710. Months of issue are January, April, July, and October. Business and Editorial Offices: 1600 John F. Kennedy Blvd., Suite 1800, Philadelphia, PA, 19103-2899. Periodicals postage paid at New York, NY and additional mailing offices. Subscription prices are $392.00 per year for US individuals, $100.00 per year for US and Canadian students/residents, $432.00 per year for Canadian individuals, $516.00 per year for international individuals, and $245.00 per year for international students/residents. For institutional access pricing please contact Customer Service via the contact information below. To receive student/resident rate, orders must be accompanied by name of affiliated institution, date of term, and the *signature* of program/residency coordinator on institution letterhead. Orders will be billed at individual rate until proof of status is received. Foreign air speed delivery is included in all *Clinics* subscription prices. All prices are subject to change without notice. **POSTMASTER:** Send address change to *Gastrointestinal Endoscopy Clinics of North America*, Elsevier Health Sciences Division, Subscription Customer Service, 3251 Riverport Lane, Maryland Heights, MO 63043. **Customer Service: 1-800-654-2452 (US). From outside the United States, call 1-314-447-8871. Fax: 1-314-447-8029. E-mail: JournalsCustomerService-usa@elsevier.com (for print support) or JournalsOnlineSupport-usa@elsevier.com (for online support).**

Reprints. For copies of 100 or more, of articles in this publication, please contact the Commercial Reprints Department, Elsevier Inc., 360 Park Avenue South, New York, NY 10010-1710. Tel. 212-633-3874; Fax: 212-633-3820; E-mail: reprints@elsevier.com.

Gastrointestinal Endoscopy Clinics of North America is covered in *Excerpta Medica, MEDLINE/PubMed (Index Medicus), and MEDLINE/MEDLARS.*

Contributors

CONSULTING EDITOR

CHARLES J. LIGHTDALE, MD
Professor of Medicine, Division of Digestive and Liver Diseases, Columbia University Medical Center, New York, New York, USA

EDITORS

KENNETH J. CHANG, MD, MASGE, FACG, AGAF, FJGES
Executive Director, Digestive Health Institute, Vincent and Anna Kong Chair in GI Endoscopic Oncology, University of California, Irvine, Irvine, California, USA

JASON B. SAMARASENA, MD, MBA, FACG, AGAF
Associate Chief, Division of Gastroenterology and Hepatology; Director, Interventional Endoscopy Training Program; Professor of Medicine, Division of Gastroenterology and Hepatology, H. H. Chao Digestive Health Institute, University of California, Irvine, Irvine, California, USA

AUTHORS

AHMAD F. ABOELEZZ, MD
Department of Internal Medicine, Gastroenterology and Hepatology Section, Faculty of Medicine, Tanta University, Tanta, Egypt

HARRY R. ASLANIAN, MD
Professor, Department of Medicine, Section of Digestive Diseases, Yale School of Medicine, New Haven, Connecticut, USA

ROSS C.D. BUERLEIN, MD
Assistant Professor of Medicine, Division of Gastroenterology and Hepatology, University of Virginia Health System, Charlottesville, Virginia, USA

ANDREW CANAKIS, DO
Fellow, Division of Gastroenterology and Hepatology, University of Maryland Medical Center, Baltimore, Maryland, USA

HYUK SOON CHOI, MD, PhD
Associate Professor, Korea University College of Medicine, Stanford University Medicine, Korea University Anam Hospital, Seoul, South Korea

FRANCES DANG, MD, MSc
University of Toronto, Toronto, Ontario, Canada

JOO HA HWANG, MD, PhD
Professor, Division of Gastroenterology and Hepatology, Department of Medicine, Stanford University Medicine, Stanford Hospital, Stanford, California, USA

SHAYAN S. IRANI, MD
Division of Gastroenterology and Hepatology, Virginia Mason Medical Center, Seattle, Washington, USA

TOUFIC KACHAAMY, MD
Chief of Medicine, Gastroenterology, City of Hope Phoenix, Arizona, USA

MOTOHIKO KATO, MD, PhD
Professor of Medicine and Director, Center for Diagnostic and Therapeutic Endoscopy, Keio University Hospital, Tokyo, Japan

MADAPPA KUNDRANDA, MD, PhD
Director, Gastrointestinal Oncology Program; Deputy Chief, Division of Medical Oncology; Adjunct Assistant Professor, Department of Gastrointestinal Medical Oncology, University of Texas MD Anderson Cancer Center, Banner MD Anderson, Gilbert, Arizona, USA

DAVID LEE, MD, MPH
Methodist Digestive Institute, Methodist Dallas Medical Center, Dallas, Texas, USA

NORIKO MATSUURA, MD
Department of Research and Development for Minimal Invasive Treatment, Cancer Center, Keio University School of Medicine, Tokyo, Japan

KINNARI MODI, MD
Resident, Department of Internal Medicine, Methodist Dallas Medical Center, Dallas, Texas, USA

MARC MONACHESE, MD, MSc
Advanced Endoscopy Fellow, University of California, Irvine - College of Medicine, Gastroenterology Fellow, University of Toronto, Trillium Health Partners, Mississauga, Ontario, Canada

THIRUVENGADAM MUNIRAJ, MD
Associate Professor, Department of Medicine, Section of Digestive Diseases, Yale School of Medicine, New Haven, Connecticut, USA

ANIL NAGAR, MD
Associate Professor, Department of Medicine, Section of Digestive Diseases, Yale School of Medicine, New Haven, Connecticut, USA

YOUSUKE NAKAI, MD, PhD
Associate Professor, Department of Gastroenterology, Graduate School of Medicine, The University of Tokyo, Tokyo, Japan; Department of Endoscopy and Endoscopic Surgery, The University of Tokyo Hospital, Bunkyo-ku, Tokyo, Japan

ATSUSHI NAKAYAMA, MD, PhD
Instructor, Department of Research and Development for Minimal Invasive Treatment, Cancer Center, Keio University School of Medicine, Tokyo, Japan

MOHAMED O. OTHMAN, MD
William T. Butler Endowed Chair for Distinguished Faculty, Department of Internal Medicine, Professor of Medicine, Gastroenterology and Hepatology Section, Baylor

College of Medicine, Chief, Gastroenterology Section at Baylor St Luke's Medical Center, Houston, Texas, USA

WOO HYUN PAIK, MD, PhD
Professor, Department of Internal Medicine, Liver Research Institute, Seoul National University Hospital, Seoul National University College of Medicine, Seoul, Korea

DO HYUN PARK, MD, PhD
Professor, Division of Gastroenterology, Department of Internal Medicine, University of Ulsan College of Medicine, Asan Medical Center, Seoul, Korea

DAVID PARSONS, MD
Instructor, Department of Medicine, Section of Digestive Diseases, Yale School of Medicine, New Haven, Connecticut, USA

JASON B. SAMARASENA, MD, MBA, FACG, AGAF
Associate Chief, Division of Gastroenterology and Hepatology; Director, Interventional Endoscopy Training Program; Professor of Medicine, Division of Gastroenterology and Hepatology, H. H. Chao Digestive Health Institute, University of California, Irvine, Irvine, California, USA

VANESSA M. SHAMI, MD, FASGE, FACG, AGAF
Professor of Medicine, Section Chief of Interventional Endoscopy, Division of Gastroenterology and Hepatology, University of Virginia Health System, Charlottesville, Virginia, USA

YOUSSEF Y. SOLIMAN, MD
Gastroenterologist, City of Hope Phoenix, Goodyear, Arizona, USA

AMIRALI TAVANGAR, MD
Division of Gastroenterology and Hepatology, Digestive Health Institute, University of California, Irvine, Irvine, California, USA

NAOHISA YAHAGI, MD, PhD
Professor of Medicine and Director, Department of Research and Development for Minimal Invasive Treatment, Cancer Center, Keio University School of Medicine, Tokyo, Japan

Contents

> White light image (WLI) findings are important for detection and characterization in the GI tract. However, magnified endoscopic examination with image enhanced endoscopy (IEE-NE) is becoming increasingly important for qualitative diagnosis of GI neoplastic lesions. IEE-ME is extremely useful for diagnosis of invasion depth in esophageal squamous cell cancer (ESCC) and colorectal cancer, whereas macroscopic findings of WLI are still useful in Barrett's adenocarcinoma (BAC) and gastric cancer. IEE-ME is also useful for diagnosis of tumor extent in BAC and gastric cancer, whereas chromoendoscopy with indigo carmine is useful in colorectal cancer and iodine staining is indispensable in ESCC.

> The last 2 decades have seen an emergence of endoscopic technologies and techniques allowing for minimally invasive modalities for assessing and sampling lesions outside of the gastrointestinal lumen, including the chest, abdomen, and pelvis. Incorporating these new endoscopic approaches has revolutionized the diagnosis and staging of extra-luminal malignancies and has enabled more accessible and safer tissue acquisition.

> The authors review the role of endoscopic ultrasound (EUS) in the staging of cancers throughout the gastrointestinal tract. EUS offers an advantage over cross-sectional imaging in locoregional tumor staging but is less sensitive in identifying distant metastasis. The addition of FNA increases diagnostic accuracy and provides a tissue diagnosis. EUS combined with cross-sectional imaging is important in accurately staging GI tumors and thereby reducing unnecessary procedures and health care costs.

Gastrointestinal cancers can have severe consequences if diagnosed at a late stage but can be cured when detected and resected at an early stage. In recent years, the significance of endoscopic screening for gastrointestinal cancers has been established, leading to the identification of early-stage cancers and precancerous lesions. Consequently, endoscopic removal of gastrointestinal tumors has emerged as an effective means of cancer treatment and prevention. This article delves into the indications, techniques, and safety measures associated with endoscopic resection of early-stage luminal cancer within the gastrointestinal tract.

Endoscopic ultrasound (EUS) has been used for various interventions to manage intra-abdominal lesions. EUS-guided antitumor therapy via delivery of chemotherapeutic agents, energy, and radioactive seeds has advantages of less invasiveness than surgical approaches, and the anatomic proximity allows easy and accurate access to the pancreas. The feasibility of EUS-guided antitumor therapy has been reported both in pancreatic solid and cystic neoplasms, with promising preliminary results. Randomized controlled trials are mandatory to further confirm its role.

 Video content accompanies this article at http://www.giendo. theclinics.com.

Endoscopic palliation of dysphagia for patients with inoperable esophageal cancer is complex, highly dependent on local expertise, and best done in a multidisciplinary fashion. Systemic therapy is the standard of care because it has been shown to improve survival. Esophageal stenting has traditionally been the most used endoscopic modality. Some modalities such as laser and photodynamic therapy are rarely used. There has been an increasing amount of data on cryotherapy, especially for patients with mild-to-moderate dysphagia on systemic chemotherapy. This article will discuss the latest evidence guiding the palliation of esophageal cancer.

Endoscopic management of gastric outlet obstruction includes balloon dilation, enteral stenting, and endoscopic ultrasound-guided gastroenterostomy (EUS-GE) to relieve mechanical blockage and reestablish per oral intake. Based on the degree of obstruction, patients may experience debilitating symptoms that can quickly lead to malnutrition and delays in chemotherapy. Compared with surgery, minimally invasive endoscopic options can provide similar clinical outcomes with fewer adverse events, faster resumption of oral feeding, and shorter hospitalizations. EUS-GE with a lumen-apposing metal stent has revolutionized treatment, especially in individuals who are not ideal surgical candidates. This article aims to describe endoscopic treatment options and future considerations.

 Video content accompanies this article at http://www.giendo. theclinics.com.

Endoscopic retrograde cholangiopancreatography (ERCP) is commonly used for managing malignant biliary obstruction; however, it is impossible if the endoscope cannot reach the ampulla of Vater, and it carries a risk of procedure-related pancreatitis. Percutaneous approach is a traditional rescue method when ERCP fails and can be useful in advanced malignant hilar biliary obstruction; however, it is invasive and carries risks of tube dislodgement, recurrent infection, and tract seeding. Endoscopic ultrasound approach may be attempted if ERCP fails and is free from the risk of pancreatitis; however, it is only possible in limited centers, and training is still difficult. Malignant biliary obstruction should be managed by leveraging the complementary strengths of these methods.

Large bowel obstruction is a serious event that occurs in approximately 25% of all intestinal obstructions. It is attributed to either benign, malignant, functional (pseudo-obstruction), or mechanical conditions. Benign etiologies of colonic obstructions include colon volvulus, anastomotic strictures, radiation injury, ischemia, inflammatory processes such as Crohn's disease, diverticulitis, bezoars, and intussusception.

Endoscopic management of gastrointestinal (GI) tumor-related bleeding is challenging for many reasons including high rebleeding rates, poor tissue response to endoscopic therapies, altered wound healing and underlying coagulopathy. However, endoscopic treatment may help reduce transfusion requirements, avoid surgery, and provide a temporary bridge to oncologic therapy. This article explores various endoscopic techniques in managing tumor bleeding from more traditional approaches of using thermal or mechanical therapy with injection therapy to newer topical agents.

The types of endoscopic interventions available for supporting the nutrition of patients with cancer have expanded in recent years to encompass a wide variety of different techniques and procedures. Many of these procedures reflect refinements of technique that have existed for some time, whereas others are implementations of novel technologies and instruments that have only become available in recent years. In this review, the authors seek to summarize the breadth of endoscopic techniques for maintaining nutrition in patients with cancer.

Amirali Tavangar and Jason B. Samarasena

The diagnosis and management of pancreatic cancer has become a standard role for the endoscopic oncologist. Pancreatic cancer can produce disabling abdominal pain, and the medical management of this pain is often challenging. Endoscopic ultrasound-guided celiac plexus neurolysis and celiac ganglia neurolysis serve as an alternative or adjunct for pain control in these patients. There remains a great deal of practice variability with regard to techniques and approaches. This article summarizes the latest scientific evidence and highlights contemporary best practice advice for these procedures.

GASTROINTESTINAL ENDOSCOPY CLINICS OF NORTH AMERICA

SERIES OF RELATED INTEREST

Gastroenterology Clinics
(www.gastro.theclinics.com)
Clinics in Liver Disease
(www.liver.theclinics.com)

THE CLINICS ARE AVAILABLE ONLINE!
Access your subscription at:
www.theclinics.com

Foreword

The Remarkably Increased Role of Gastrointestinal Endsocopy in Oncology

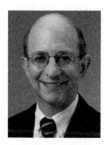

Charles J. Lightdale, MD
Consulting Editor

Yes, it is not far-fetched to consider the concept of an endoscopic oncologist, the subject of this issue of the *Gastrointestinal Endoscopy Clinics of North America*. Endoscopists have become increasingly involved in the multidisciplinary management of cancer patients. Certainly, the role of endoscopists in prevention, diagnosis, treatment, and palliation of cancers involving both luminal and solid gastrointestinal organs has grown remarkably over the past three decades, as brilliantly presented by the Editors for this issue of the *Gastrointestinal Endoscopy Clinics of North America*, Dr Kenneth J. Chang and Dr Jason B. Samarasena. They have assembled an extraordinary international group of authors covering the entire spectrum of endoscopic applications related to oncology. Don't miss this terrific issue.

As an addendum, this will be my last issue as Consulting Editor of the *Gastrointestinal Endoscopy Clinics of North America*, as I have decided to retire from the position that I have held for 25 years. I have immensely enjoyed my role in choosing guest editors and topics and helping to shepherd so many great issues during this time. I was very fortunate that my tenure coincided with amazing growth and progress in gastrointestinal endoscopy benefiting millions of patients. I was aided enormously by the very professional staff at Elsevier. In particular, I will be forever grateful to Senior Editor Kerry Holland, who has worked with me from the beginning, always providing friendly, sound advice and steady guidance. While it was time for me to let go of the wheel, I feel doubly fortunate that the new Consulting Editor will be Dr Ashley Faulx. She has a broad knowledge of the field and is widely recognized as a thought leader, and I am certain she will be successful and bring new perspectives to the role.

Gastrointest Endoscopy Clin N Am 34 (2024) xiii–xiv
https://doi.org/10.1016/j.giec.2023.08.002
1052-5157/24/© 2023 Published by Elsevier Inc.

giendo.theclinics.com

The inherent strength of the endoscopic method will persist; new developments will come at a rapid pace, and I fully expect that the *Gastrointestinal Endoscopy Clinics of North America* will continue to thrive.

Charles J. Lightdale, MD
Department of Medicine
Columbia University Medical Center
161 Fort Washington Avenue
New York, NY 10032, USA

E-mail address:
CJL18@columbia.edu

Preface

The Vital Role of the Endoscopic Oncologist

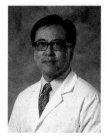
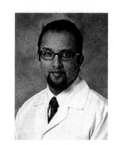

Kenneth J. Chang, MD, MASGE, FACG, AGAF, FJGES

Jason B. Samarasena, MD, MBA, FACG, AGAF

Editors

A HISTORICAL PERSPECTIVE

In 1993, I was recruited to be the Head of Gastrointestinal Oncology at the University of California, Irvine within our new NCI-designated Comprehensive Cancer Center. Prior to accepting this position, I interviewed a few prominent figures who worked in this unique space where gastrointestinal (GI) intersects with Oncology—and I came to the conclusion that this was indeed an area of clinically unmet needs. This was further confirmed by my father's diagnosis of locally advanced colon cancer and the journey we would travel together as a family. This was the era where the gastroenterologist was making the diagnosis of various digestive cancers, but would then quickly send the patient off to the medical oncologist without much further involvement or input. The medical oncologist, on the other hand, would render chemotherapy with or without radiation, yet may not have the full understanding and command of the GI issues that might arise during and after treatment. So, armed with an endoscope and the relatively new technology called endoscopic ultrasound (EUS), I stepped into a position that I knew relatively little about. Having my new professional home embedded in a Cancer Center, where my neighbors were medical, radiation, gynecologic, and surgical oncologists, I began discovering the vital role that the GI Endoscopic Oncologist would and could play. I soon started an advanced fellowship in EUS and GI Oncology to train those of like mind, and years later I received the first endowed chair bearing this very title, "The Vincent and Anna Kong Chair of Gastrointestinal Endoscopic Oncology."

Gastrointest Endoscopy Clin N Am 34 (2024) xv–xviii
https://doi.org/10.1016/j.giec.2023.08.001
1052-5157/24/© 2023 Published by Elsevier Inc.

giendo.theclinics.com

THE VITAL ROLE OF THE GASTROINTESTINAL ENDOSCOPIC ONCOLOGIST

Over the past three decades, the role of the GI Endoscopic Oncologist has emerged and expanded. In these 12 articles, we have invited internationally renowned Endoscopic Oncologists to review and update all the exciting growth areas. **Table 1** summarizes the specific roles of the Endoscopic Oncologist and how we've evolved over three decades. Endoscopic detection of superficial GI cancer and the ability to assess submucosal invasion by leveraging image-enhanced and magnifying endoscopy have improved dramatically ("Endoscopic Diagnosis of Superficial Gastrointestinal Cancer by Yahagi). The power of EUS in detecting and diagnosing tumors located adjacent to the GI tract, including the posterior mediastinum, lung, peritoneum, and liver; and the complementary roles of EUS, Endoscopic Retrograde Cholangiopancreatography, and Cholangioscopy for biliary cancer, has become standard of care ("Endoscopic Diagnosis of Extraluminal Cancer" by Shami and Buerlein). EUS for cancer staging has become more complementary to computed tomography (CT)/MRI as imaging has improved significantly, although definitive N staging with EUS–fine needle aspiration (FNA)/biopsy has unique clinical value (Endoscopic Ultrasound Cancer Staging" by Aslanian and colleagues). Endoscopic resection for early cancer, while in its infancy in the early 1990s, has become mainstream and indispensable with the expanding role of Endoscopic Mucosal Resection, Endoscopic Submucosal Dissection, Endoscopic Full-Thickness Resection, and Submucosal Tunneling Endoscopic Resection ("Endoscopic Resection for Early Cancer" by Hwang and Choi). EUS-guided delivery of antitumor agents, first reported in 2000, has included injection, ablation, and radioactive seed implantation for both solid and cystic pancreatic tumors. Its definitive role in the treatment of neuroendocrine tumors and its adjunctive/immunomodulatory strategy in pancreatic cancer still await confirmatory clinical trials ("EUS-guided Antitumor Therapy" by Nakai). Working collaboratively with the entire Oncology community, the Endoscopic Oncologist is called on to help patients suffering from luminal obstruction from a wide variety of primary cancers. Whether its esophageal ("Endoscopic Palliative Therapies for Esophageal Cancer" by Soliman and colleagues), gastric ("Endoscopic Treatment of Gastric Outlet Obstruction" by Canakis and Irani), biliary ("Endoscopic Management of Malignant Biliary Obstruction" by Paik and Park), or colonic ("Endoscopic Management of Colonic Obstruction" by Othman) obstruction, we are uniquely resourced with self-expanding stents, lumen apposing stents, and ablation therapies; to either bridge or completely bypass the site of malignant stricture. Palliative treatment also includes cessation of tumor bleeding ("Endoscopic Management of Tumor Bleeding: Techniques and Strategies" by Monachese and Dang) and pain management with EUS-guided celiac plexus and celiac ganglion neurolysis ("Endoscopic Ultrasound Guided Pain Management" by Samarasena). Finally, critically important to all cancer patients is the need for enteral feeding when oral intake is compromised ("Endoscopic Nutrition of Cancer Patients" by Lee). We hope that by reviewing the

Table 1
The endoscopic oncologist's toolbox - 30 years later

The Role of the Endoscopic Oncologist	1993	2023
Diagnosing luminal cancers	Low-quality imaging, biopsy with forceps, histology only	High-quality imaging, image enhancement, magnifying endoscopy, high-yield sampling, biological markers
Diagnosing extraluminal cancers	CT was at its infancy; MRI was not yet available. EUS emerged to image and biopsy pancreatic, liver, biliary, adrenal, and lung cancers	EUS, especially with FNA/fine needle biopsy, is complementary to CT/MRI. EUS, endoscopic retrograde cholangiopancreatography, and cholangioscopy are complementary to imaging for biliary cancer
Staging GI and other cancers	EUS was more accurate than CT for staging esophageal, gastric, pancreatic, and rectal cancers	CT/MRI imaging has improved, so less need for EUS staging, although complementary; EUS/FNA for nodal staging is valuable
Endoscopic resection of early cancer	Endoscopic mucosal resection started in Japan and was just making its way to the West	EMR, ESD, EFTR, and STER have become mainstream in the West and indispensable for early cancer treatment
Endoscopic delivery of antitumor agents	Early case reports of delivering agents via EUS-guided fine needle injection	Expanded to include injection, ablation, and radioactive seed implantation for both solid and cystic pancreatic tumors
Endoscopic treatment of luminal (esophageal, gastric, colonic, biliary) obstruction	Dilation, alcohol injection, ND:YAG laser, early stiff stents, venting G-tube	Softer, fully and partially covered stents, lumen-opposing stents, gastrojejunostomy, hepaticojejunostomy, choledochojejunostomy, cholecystojejunostomy, and similar
Endoscopic management of tumor bleeding	ND:YAG laser, alcohol injection	Argon plasma coagulation, topical hemostatic agents
Endoscopic pain management	EUS-guided celiac neurolysis	EUS-guided celiac ganglion lysis; pancreatic duct stenting
Endoscopic nutritional support	G-tube	G-J tube, direct J-tube, luminal stenting and bypass

Abbreviations: EFTR, endoscopic full thickness resection; EMR, endoscopic mucosal resection; ESD, endoscopic submucosal dissection; STER, submucosal tunneling endoscopic resection.

past, present, and future role of the Endoscopic Oncologist, we can inspire the next generation to multiply the impact to those in need of our skills.

Kenneth J. Chang, MD, MASGE, FACG, AGAF, FJGES
University of California, Irvine
Digestive Health Institute
Building 22C, 3rd Floor, RT 99, Room 106
101 The City Drive
Orange, CA 92868, USA

Jason B. Samarasena, MD, MBA, FACG, AGAF
University of California, Irvine
Irvine, CA, USA

E-mail addresses:
kchang@uci.edu (K.J. Chang)
jsamaras@hs.uci.edu (J.B. Samarasena)

Endoscopic Diagnosis of Superficial Gastrointestinal Cancer

Atsushi Nakayama, MD, PhD[a], Motohiko Kato, MD, PhD[b],
Noriko Matsuura, MD[a], Naohisa Yahagi, MD, PhD[a,*]

KEYWORDS

- Endoscopic diagnosis
- Magnified endoscopic examination with image-enhanced endoscopy (IEE-ME)
- Esophageal squamous cell cancer (ESCC) • Barrett's adenocarcinoma (BAC)
- Gastric cancer • Colorectal cancer

KEY POINTS

- White light image findings are still important for detection and characterization of early neoplastic lesions in the gastrointestinal tract.
- The macroscopic type classification based on the Paris classification is important for diagnosis of superficial gastrointestinal neoplastic lesions.
- IEE-ME is becoming increasingly important and is quite useful for qualitative diagnosis of gastrointestinal neoplastic lesions.
- Different diagnostic modalities should be selected depending on each organ for the diagnosis of invasion depth and tumor extent.

INTRODUCTION

Early neoplastic lesions in the gastrointestinal tract (GI) can be broadly classified into macroscopic types (Type 0) (**Fig. 1**) based on the Paris classification,[1] and the diagnosis of invasion depth can be predicted to some extent for each of these macroscopic types. In addition, image-enhanced endoscopy (IEE), described below, may be used to assist in the diagnosis of the presence and invasion depth of the lesion. The main importance of accurately diagnosing these endoscopic findings is to evaluate the presence or absence of submucosal (SM) invasion, since it determines the treatment

[a] Department of Research and Development for Minimal Invasive Treatment, Cancer Center, Keio University School of Medicine, 35 Shinanomachi, Shinjuku-ku, Tokyo 160-8582, Japan;
[b] Center for Diagnostic and Therapeutic Endoscopy, Keio University Hospital, 35 Shinanomachi, Shinjuku-ku, Tokyo 160-8582, Japan
* Corresponding author. Department of Research and Development for Minimal Invasive Treatment, Cancer Center, Keio University School of Medicine, 35 Shinanomachi, Shinjuku-ku, Tokyo 160-8582, Japan.
E-mail address: yahagi-tky@umin.ac.jp

Gastrointest Endoscopy Clin N Am 34 (2024) 1–17
https://doi.org/10.1016/j.giec.2023.08.003
1052-5157/24/© 2023 Elsevier Inc. All rights reserved.
giendo.theclinics.com

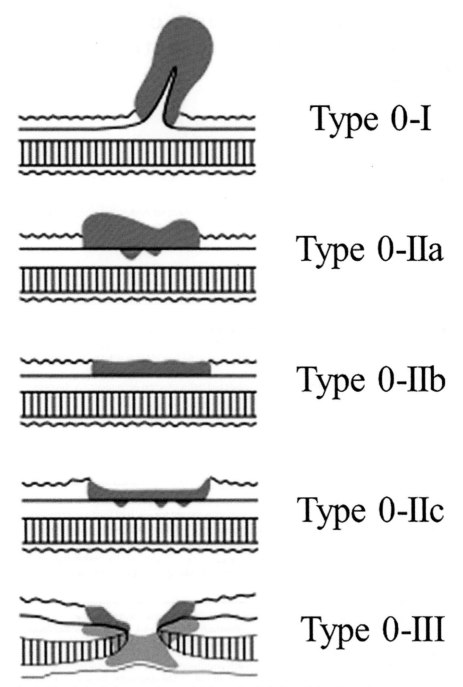

Type 0-I

Type 0-IIa

Type 0-IIb

Type 0-IIc

Type 0-III

Fig. 1. Morphological types of superficial neoplastic lesion of the GI tract.

strategy (mainly endoscopic or surgical) for early-stage neoplastic lesions of the GI tract. Based on this principle, we discuss the endoscopic diagnosis of superficial neoplastic lesions in the esophagus, stomach, and colorectum, including (1) detection, (2) differentiation, (3) invasion depth, (4) lateral extent, (5) magnified endoscopic examination with IEE (IEE-ME) (only esophageal squamous cell carcinoma and colorectal cancer are explained independently), and (6) treatment strategy for each target lesion.

ESOPHAGEAL CANCER
Esophageal Squamous Cell Carcinoma

Detection
Because drinking and smoking habits are risk factors for esophageal squamous cell carcinoma (ESCC), especially in those cases, one should attempt to recognize superficial cancer by noting a change in color tone such as redness, and a slight depression or elevation during white-light observation. IEE can more easily detect suspicious lesions as brownish areas and can be used in conjunction with white light imaging (WLI) as appropriate.[2] Iodine staining is also very useful for detection as it shows a regional zone of unstained mucosa. In addition, typical ESCC usually turns pinkish in the iodine unstained areas a few minutes after iodine staining. This is called the "pink color sign" and is considered a characteristic finding of ESCC.[3]

Differentiation
Most ESCCs, especially early-stage lesions, show the so-called differentiated type histopathologically. Therefore, the following endoscopic diagnosis is basically related to differentiated squamous cell carcinoma.

Invasion depth
The frequency of lymph node metastasis in ESCC correlates with the depth of the tumor; thus, accurate diagnosis of invasion depth is important in determining the treatment strategy. Because esophageal cancer is more invasive than gastric and colorectal cancer, it should be diagnosed more carefully.

ESCC originates from the epithelium (EP), extends to the lamina propria mucosae (LPM), and then progressively further invades to the muscularis mucosae (MM), the shallow SM layer (SM1: up to 200 μm), and the deep SM layer (SM2: deeper than 200 μm). In general, lesions up to LPM are good candidates for endoscopic treatment, but deeply SM invasive carcinoma is not indicated for endoscopic treatment because of the extremely high risk of lymph node metastasis. Invasion depth of most ESCCs less than 2 cm in diameter is up to T1a-LPM; however, the invasion depth of ESCCs is often estimated by referring to the macroscopic type of the lesion as follows[4] **(Fig. 2)**. In addition, the minimal change in shape associated with insufflation and deflation is a characteristic of deeply invasive cancer.

Type 0-I. Generally, Type 0-I is interpreted as a finding that suggests SM invasion.

Type 0-IIa. Most lesions are whitish or isochromatic, and the height of the elevation and the size of the granules in the granular lesions should be noted. In other words, lesions up to T1a-LPM have a relatively low height (1–2 mm) and no or minimal granular changes (1–2 mm). On the other hand, T1a-MM/T1b-SM1 cancers are more erythematous and nodular in shape, with elevations exceeding 1 to 2 mm in height.

Type 0-IIb. Type 0-IIb is usually found incidentally as reddish area in WLI, brownish area in IEE-ME, and unstained area in iodine staining within completely flat mucosa. It is generally supposed to be superficial lesions such as T1a-EP/LPM cancers.

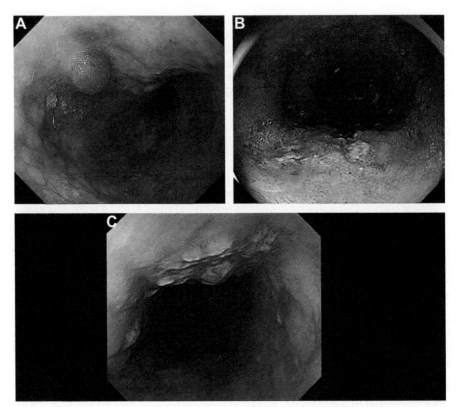

Fig. 2. Endoscopic findings suggestive of SM invasion of esophageal squamous cell carcinoma. (*A*) Type 0-I component. (*B*) Apparent granular changes within Type 0-IIa. (*C*) Strong irregularity of depressed surface with Type 0-IIc.

Type 0-IIc. Type 0-IIc is characterized by a mildly erythematous depression and is the most frequent grossly visible form of ESCC. Shallow flat depression usually suggests T1a-EP/LPM cancers, whereas more irregular concavity and convexity within the depression suggests T1a-MM/T1b-SM1 cancers.

Type 0-III. Type 0-III is a more deeply recessed lesion than Type 0-IIc, and together with Type 0-I, it is a grossly visible type that is reminiscent of deep SM invasion.

Although endoscopic ultrasound sonography (EUS) is sometimes used as an adjunctive diagnosis for invasion depth of GI cancers, it has been reported that EUS may increase overdiagnosis in ESCC compared with WLI findings or IEE-ME.[5]

Lateral extent
As mentioned in the section on detection, ESCC is often difficult to detect with WLI alone, and the entire lesion is more easily observed with IEE[2] or iodine staining.[3] IEE is an important modality because it can contribute to qualitative diagnosis as well as the diagnosis of invasion depth. However, it is sometimes difficult to determine the exact extent of the lesion by itself. Therefore, iodine staining is indispensable and the most useful modality for the diagnosis of tumor extent especially before endoscopic resection although it is sometimes unpleasant stimulus to the patients.

The magnified endoscopic classification of the Japan Esophageal Society

IEE-ME assists in the qualitative diagnosis of ESCC by evaluating the intrapapillary capillary loop (IPCL) in the superficial layers of the tumor.[6] It is thought to reflect the degree of histologic atypia, since the morphology of the IPCL changes according to histologic structure. The following is an introduction of the magnified endoscopic classification of the Japan Esophageal Society (**Fig. 3**).[7]

Type A. No or minimal changes in IPCL.

Type B. Type B is defined as having severe changes in vascular morphology and is subdivided into the following 3 categories.

   B1: Loop-like abnormal vessels that are dilated, tortuous, of unequal caliber, and of uneven shape suggesting T1a-EP/LPM.

   B2: Abnormal vessels with poor loop formation suggesting T1a-MM/T1b-SM1.

   B3: Highly dilated, irregular vessels (more than 3 times as large as B2 vessels and with an irregular vessel diameter >60 µm) suggesting T1b-SM2.

   Type A vessels are seen in lesions with inflammation or low-grade atypia and are acceptable for follow-up.

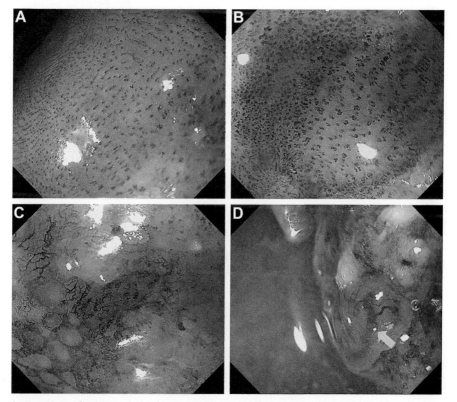

Fig. 3. IEE-ME findings of esophageal squamous cell carcinoma (classification by the Japan Esophageal Society). (*A*) Slight change in vascular morphology (sparse and faint dot-shaped capillary loop) (Type A). (*B*) Loop-like abnormal vessels that are dilated, tortuous, of unequal caliber, and of unequal shape (Type 2A). (*C*) Anomalous vessels with poor loop formation (Type 2B). (*D*) Highly dilated irregular vessels (*arrow*, Type B3) IEE-ME, magnified endoscopic examination with image-enhanced endoscopy.

Type B vessels are considered ESCC and should be treated. Type B1 and B2 vessels are differentiated by the presence or absence of loop-like structures. Here, we present a typical case of ESCC with Type B1 vessels (**Fig. 4**).

Treatment strategy for superficial esophageal squamous cell carcinoma based on endoscopic findings

According to the Japanese guidelines for esophageal cancer, T1a-EP/LPM cancer is an absolute indication for endoscopic treatment, T1a-MM/T1b-SM1 cancer is a relative indication for endoscopic treatment in the absence of metastasis, and T1b-SM2 or deeper cancer is an indication for surgical treatment.[8] The final treatment plan must be based on a comprehensive judgment in conjunction with the WLI findings and computed tomography (CT) findings.

Barrett's Adenocarcinoma

Definition and diagnosis of Barrett's epithelium

Barrett's adenocarcinoma (BAC) is a malignant tumor that originates from Barrett's EP. Therefore, we will first discuss the definition and diagnosis of Barrett's EP.

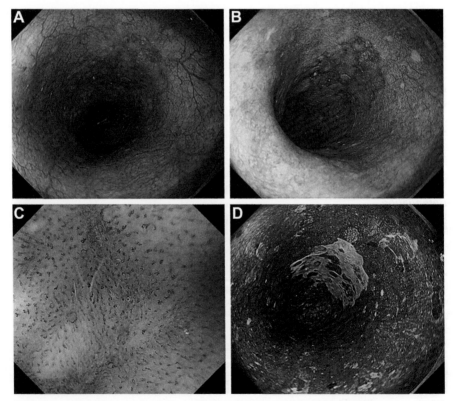

Fig. 4. Typical endoscopic findings of esophageal squamous cell carcinoma. (*A*) A 20 mm Type 0-IIc tumor with a mild erythematous tone was seen on the anterior wall of the lower cancers. (*B*) IEE showed brownish area. (*C*) IEE-ME showed a Type B1 vessel of the magnified endoscopic classification of the Japan Esophageal Society. (*D*) Iodine staining showed a well-defined tumor and the pink color sign was slightly positive. IEE, image-enhanced endoscopy; IEE-ME, magnified endoscopic examination with image-enhanced endoscopy.

Barrett's EP is defined as a continuous columnar epithelial growth of the mucosa of the lower esophagus from the stomach. To diagnose it endoscopically, the esophago-gastric junction (EGJ) must be identified. In Japan, the EGJ is defined as the lower end of the fenestra of the lower esophagus on endoscopy, or the proximal end of the longitudinal folds of the stomach if the fenestra cannot be identified.[9] On the other hand, in Europe and the United States, the EGJ is defined primarily as the upper margin of the gastric mucosal folds.[10] Despite these differences, the diagnosis of Barrett's EP is easy once the EGJ is identified. In addition, the Prague criteria are often used to classify Barrett's EP.[11] This involves measuring the circumferential extent (C (cm)) of Barrett's EP from the EGJ and the maximum length (M (cm)) of the lingual portion extending from it (eg, C2M4).[11]

Detection
In Europe and the United States, endoscopic resection is recommended when BAC is histologically diagnosed by random biopsy as recommended in the American Collage of Gastroenterology (ACG) guidelines or when mucosal irregularities are present.[10] On the other hand, targeted biopsy based on endoscopic findings has been reported as an effective alternative to random biopsy, and a meta-analysis conducted by American Society for Gastrointestinal Endoscopy (ASGE) reported that target biopsy based on endoscopic findings is a potential alternative to conventional random biopsy.[12] Therefore, it is expected that target biopsy from the site of abnormal endoscopic findings will become more important than random biopsy in Europe and the United States. Meanwhile, in Japan, BAC is often endoscopically diagnosed in accordance with gastric cancer because it is composed of columnar EP same as the stomach. In particular, it is important to focus on redness within Barrett's EP, as it is often the trigger for BAC identification. In IEE-ME, the diagnosis is made by evaluating the microsurface and microvascular pattern of the EP as either regular or irregular, based on the diagnostic criteria for gastric cancer[13] described below. If both are determined to be regular, the lesion is judged as noncancer; otherwise, the other lesion is judged as BAC.[14] Here we have a typical case of BAC diagnosed by irregularities in both the microsurface and microvascular pattern (**Fig. 5**).

Differentiation
Because most BAC is a differentiated-type carcinoma, the diagnosis regarding differentiated-type adenocarcinoma (histopathologically well to moderately differentiated tubular adenocarcinoma) is described below.

Invasion depth
Although no unique diagnostic criteria have been established for the invasion depth diagnosis of BAC due to its anatomic characteristics and frequency, in Japan, the diagnosis is often made in accordance with that of gastric cancer, which is discussed below. In other words, the diagnosis is based on macroscopic findings, and unlike ESCC and colorectal cancer, IEE-ME is considered to be only a qualitative diagnosis including a diagnosis of tumor extent. Note that in Barrett's mucosa, the muscularis mucosae are doubled, and the invasion depth may be determined to be slightly shallower than that of ESCC.

Regarding diagnosis of invasion depth by EUS, the EGJ is reported to have a lower rate of accuracy than the esophagus[15,16]; therefore, it is not recommended to perform it routinely.

Lateral extent
BAC is often recognized as reddish Type 0-IIa or IIc; however, the diagnosis of tumor extent may be difficult in tumors with a long segment Barrett's esophagus background

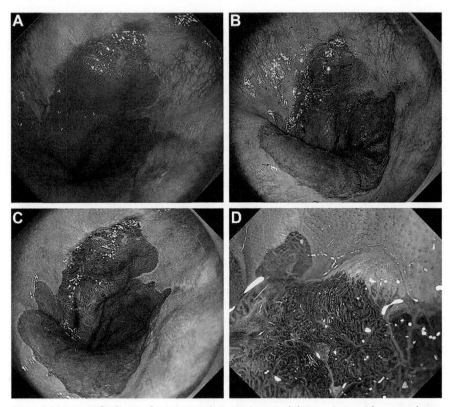

Fig. 5. Endoscopic findings of Barrett's adenocarcinoma. (*A*) Type 0-IIa with an erythematous tone in Barrett's epithelium on the antero-dorsal wall of the esophagogastric junction. (*B*) Indigo carmine spraying enhanced the irregularity of the lesion and clarified its extent. (*C*) IEE revealed the entire lesion as a rough area due to the irregular surface structure. (*D*) IEE-ME showed regional vascular irregularities and structural irregularities. IEE, image-enhanced endoscopy; IEE-ME, magnified endoscopic examination with image-enhanced endoscopy.

due to Type 0-IIb extension. A more detailed diagnosis of extent is made based on chromoendoscopy with indigo carmine and IEE-ME findings,[14] and biopsy may be performed if necessary.

Treatment strategy for superficial Barrett's adenocarcinoma based on endoscopic findings
Endoscopic treatment of BAC is performed in accordance with ESCC, and is indicated for patients with previously diagnosed cT1a carcinoma.[17]

GASTRIC CANCER
Detection

It is important to observe the stomach systematically and efficiently, paying attention to changes in coloration and surface irregularities. In patients with *Helicobacter pylori (Hp)* infection or a history of *Hp* infection, careful observation should be made to avoid overlooking differentiated-type carcinoma by paying attention to slight changes in the mucosa, focusing on the atrophic mucosa and its bordering areas. Undifferentiated-as well as differentiated-type carcinoma may occur in *Hp* uninfected patients, although less frequently than in *Hp*-infected patients, and particularly a slightly whitish change should be focused. If gastric cancer is suspected by WLI, microsurface and microvascular pattern are evaluated by IEE-ME and if both are determined to be regular, the lesion is diagnosed as noncancer; otherwise, the lesion is diagnosed as gastric cancer (MESDA-G).[13]

Differentiation

Gastric cancer can be classified into 2 types based on histology: differentiated-type carcinoma (well to moderately differentiated tubular adenocarcinoma) and undifferentiated-type carcinoma (poorly differentiated adenocarcinoma including signet-ring cell carcinoma). Although histologic type can often be inferred from the background mucosa and the endoscopic findings, histologic evaluation is indispensable because it is necessary to determine the treatment strategy described below. In gastric cancer, the shape of the microvascular architecture is the focus of qualitative evaluation. Differentiated-type carcinomas that develop mainly in the setting of *Hp* infection-associated atrophic gastritis often show a fine network pattern, whereas undifferentiated-type carcinomas show a corkscrew pattern (**Fig. 6**).[18] The estimation of gastric cancer differentiation by IEE-ME is useful for small lesions; however, it is sometimes difficult to determine the degree of differentiation for larger lesions because it is difficult to observe the entire lesion in detail and various histologic types may coexist. Targeted biopsy should be taken to confirm histology in gastric cancer since treatment strategy is different depending on differentiation.

Invasion depth

Because the invasion depth of gastric cancer cannot be diagnosed by IEE-ME, information from the macroscopic findings by WLI is important (**Fig. 7**).[19]

Type 0-I
If the tumor is less than 2 cm, it is generally an T1a (M) cancer. If the tumor is more than 2 cm in diameter and has a broad base or is accompanied by a depression on the tumor surface, T1b (SM) cancer is suspected. If the tumor is more than 3 cm in diameter, it is more likely to be deeply invasive SM cancer.

Type 0-IIa
If the tumor has a smooth surface or is relatively large but has no irregularities in lobular structure, it is likely to be an T1a (M) cancer regardless of size. T1b (SM) cancer is suspected when the nodules are irregularly sized, markedly erythematous or coarsely structured.

Type 0-IIb
Type 0-IIb is usually found incidentally as a discolored area and is generally T1a (M) cancer.

Type 0-IIc
Majority of small flat depressed lesions are T1a (M) cancer; however, T1b (SM) cancer is suspected in the following cases.

- Marked redness of the depressed surface
- Remarkable depressed surface, nodules of unequal size, unstructured
- Stiffening of the wall
- Lesion diameter > 2 cm
- Raised margins of the lesion (SM tumor-like elevation)

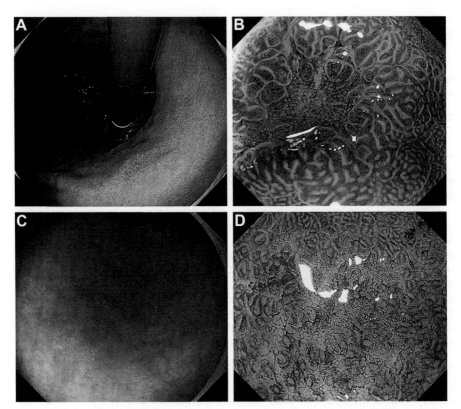

Fig. 6. Typical endoscopic findings of gastric cancer according to degree of differentiation. (*A*) Type 0-IIc lesion (well-differentiated tubular adenocarcinoma) of 5 mm in diameter was found in the lesser curvature of the middle gastric corpus. (*B*) IEE-ME findings in (*A*). Irregular microsurface pattern and irregular microvascular pattern with a demarcation line were observed. (*C*) Type 0-IIc lesion (poorly differentiated adenocarcinoma) of 15 mm in diameter was found in the greater curvature of the gastric antrum. (*D*) IEE-ME findings in (*C*). Absent microsurface pattern and irregular microvascular pattern with a demarcation line were observed. Microvascular structure showed as corkscrew-shaped. IEE-ME, magnified endoscopic examination with image-enhanced endoscopy.

Type 0-IIc with ulceration

This type is the most difficult to diagnose in terms of depth. In particular, the erythema, stiffening of the wall, and marginal elevation can be explained by ulceration (UL), and are not immediately indicative of T1b (SM) cancer. As a general rule, if there is no evidence of remarkable depression, nodules of unequal size, or unstructured surface it is often interpreted as T1a (M) cancer with UL.

Type 0-III

Pure Type 0-III is rare and difficult to diagnose in detail because the base of the ulcer is covered with white moss. Therefore, it is important to reexamine the ulcer after treatment with acid suppressant to evaluate for the presence of a Type 0-IIc component at the ulcer margins.

Moreover, it has been reported that EUS is useful in the diagnosis of invasion depth in gastric cancer as for differentiated-type carcinomas and lesions that are judged to be low-confidence SM cancer based on WLI findings alone.[20,21]

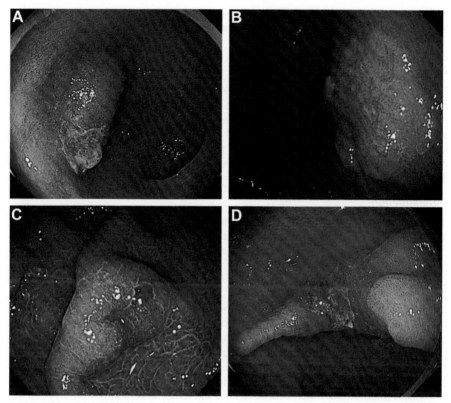

Fig. 7. Endoscopic findings suggestive of SM invasion of gastric cancer. (*A*) Type 0-I lesion over 3 cm. (*B*) Type 0-IIa lesion with apparent erythema and rough surface texture. (*C*) Type 0-IIc lesion with a submucosal tumor-like elevation. (*D*) Type 0-IIc lesion with fold convergence and thickening of the recessed surface.

Lateral extent

Initially, a qualitative diagnosis of the lesion is made by recognizing the protrusions, depressions, differences in color tone, and changes in the surface structure of the mucosa on the tumor by WLI. Then, indigo carmine is sprayed to diagnose the extent of the lesion. However, especially if the lesion is Type 0-IIb or if the background mucosa is strongly atrophic after *Hp* eradication, it may be difficult to accurately diagnose the extent of the lesion based on WLI findings alone. Therefore, IEE-ME can be used in combination with WLI for a more detailed diagnosis of the extent. The microsurface and microvascular pattern are evaluated and when a demarcation line consisting of areas where either one or both are irregular is observed, a diagnosis of tumor extent can be made[22] (see **Fig. 6**).

Treatment Strategy for Gastric Cancer Based on Endoscopic Findings

The latest Japanese guidelines for the treatment of gastric cancer define the indications according to the differentiation of the cancers. Namely, (1) for differentiated-type adenocarcinoma, lesions judged to be T1a (M) have no size limit, but lesions with UL must be less than 3 cm, and (2) for undifferentiated-type adenocarcinoma, lesions less than 2 cm without UL are indicated for endoscopic treatment.[23] The indication for endoscopic treatment should be carefully determined based on the WLI and IEE-ME findings described above together with CT findings.

COLORECTAL CANCER
Detection

To detect colorectal tumors including carcinoma, it is necessary to increase the adenoma detection rate (ADR) by adjusting the air volume around the flexure or by reciprocating observation using WLI. It has been reported that ADR can be improved by using various modalities available today,[24] and it is important to improve the quality of colonoscopy, since it has been reported that improving ADR not only leads to early detection of colorectal cancer, but also reduces the risk of death from colorectal cancer.[25]

Differentiation

The majority of colorectal cancers are differentiated-type adenocarcinomas arising from adenoma-carcinoma sequences,[26] and other well-known types are *de novo* carcinomas[27] and those arising from sessile serrated lesions,[28] most of them are differentiated adenocarcinomas.

Invasion Depth

In recent years, the indication for endoscopic treatment of early-stage colorectal cancer has been gradually expanding. According to the Japanese colorectal cancer treatment guidelines, T1a (SM1) cancer, which is considered to have a very low risk of lymph node metastasis, is defined as cancer up to 1000 μm from the bottom end of muscularis mucosae.[29] This means that endoscopic diagnosis of deep-invasive cancer with SM > 1000 μm (T1b) is important for subsequent treatment decisions.

In colon and rectum, macroscopic type of the tumor is very important to estimate the risk of SM invasion. Laterally spreading tumor (LST) is frequently used as a colloquial term for colorectal tumors characterized by horizontal growth and extension that are 10 mm or more in diameter.[30] LST is divided into granular type and nongranular type. The former is further divided into homogeneous type (LST-G (H)) and nodular mixed type (LST-G (M)), whereas the latter is divided into flat type (LST-NG (F)) and pseudo-depressed type (LST-NG (PD)) (**Fig. 8**). LST-G (H) has almost no SM cancer, even when the tumor size is large, whereas LST-G (M) has some risk of SM cancer. LST-NG (F) is considered to have a relatively low cancer-bearing rate, but the risk of SM invasion is increased in large lesions.

In addition, important endoscopic findings suggestive of deep SM invasive cancer are (1) tautness, (2) deep depression, (3) irregularity of the depressed area, and (4) fold formation (**Fig. 9**).[31] For colorectal lesions, pit pattern classification was the gold standard that can be used not only for qualitative diagnosis but also as an indicator for depth diagnosis,[32] and widely used in Japan until recently. However, currently there is a tendency to refrain from using it because of the potential risk of carcinogenesis

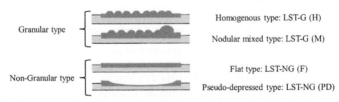

Fig. 8. Macroscopic type classification of lateral spreading tumors in the colorectum.

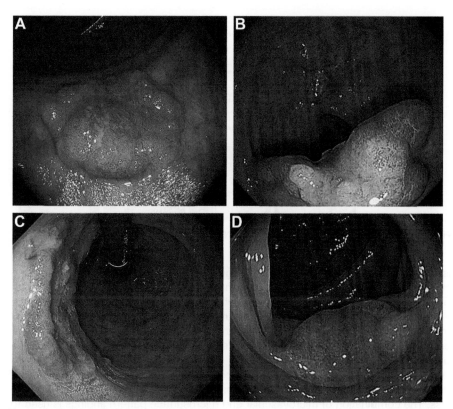

Fig. 9. Endoscopic findings suggestive of SM invasion of colorectal cancer. (*A*) Protruded component with an appearance of fullness. (*B*) Deep concavity. (*C*) Stiff and irregularly depressed area. (*D*) Convergence of folds.

of crystal violet.[33] Furthermore, it should be remembered that the pit pattern classification is a diagnostic tool only for colorectal tumors and should not be used for other GI tumors.

If the above-mentioned WLI findings alone are not sufficient to make a diagnosis of invasion depth, EUS can be used as an adjunctive diagnostic tool. In particular, EUS has been reported to be useful in diagnosing the SM cancer, especially in superficial flat-type tumors including LSTs.[34]

Lateral Extent

Indigocarmine spraying may enhance irregularities within the lesion and aid in extent diagnosis; however, in general, colorectal cancer is often relatively easy to diagnose the tumor extent.

Japan NBI Expert Team Classification

The Japan NBI Expert Team (JNET) classification is gaining importance in the qualitative diagnosis of colorectal tumors, replacing the pit pattern classification, and is attracting attention because it is simple, does not use any stains, and has high diagnostic accuracy, as it uses IEE-ME to evaluate microvascular and microsurface patterns[35](**Fig. 10**). The microvascular pattern is thin and sparse in normal mucosa and hyperplastic lesions and is difficult to visualize, but in tumors, the vascular pattern

	Type 1	Type 2A	Type 2B	Type 3
Vessel pattern	Invisible	Regular caliber Regular distribution (meshed/spiral pattern)	Variable caliber Irregular distribution	Loose vessel areas Interruption of thick vessels
Surface pattern	Regular dark or white spots Similar to surrounding normal mucosa	Regular (tubular/branched/papillary)	Irregular or obscure	Amorphous areas
Most likely histology	Hyperplastic polyp/ Sessile serrated lesion	Low grade intramucosal neoplasia	High grade intramucosal neoplasia/Shallow submucosal invasive cancer	Deep submucosal invasive cancer
Endoscopic image				

Fig. 10. Summary of The JNET classification. JNET, Japan NBI expert team.

is a brownish color due to renewed angiogenesis, increased vascular diameter, and increased vascular density. In adenomas, they are observed in a well-defined reticular pattern, whereas in cancers, there is heterogeneity of vessel diameter, irregular vascular running, and disorganized distribution caused by invasive growth and stromal reaction, and in deep SM invasive cancers, fragmented vessels and avascular areas are observed. The microsurface pattern reflects the combined structure of the pit orifice and the marginal EP of the fossa, which appears white and devoid of blood vessels. In cancer, it appears irregular, reflecting the structural atypia of the glandular ducts, and when the ducts are severely destroyed by invasion, it appears structureless. The combination of microvascular and microsurface pattern findings is used to classify and diagnose as Type 1 (normal, hyperplastic, and sessile serrated lesions), Type 2A (adenoma to intramucosal cancer), Type 2B (intramucosal cancer to SM slightly invasive cancer), and Type 3 (SM highly invasive cancer). In the JNET classification, vascular and surface patterns are diagnosed on the basis of "or" rather than "and," and findings of either one or the other are used to classify the lesion into the corresponding category.

Treatment Strategy for Colorectal Cancer Based on Endoscopic Findings

The indication for endoscopic treatment of colorectal cancer does not depend on the size or macroscopic type of the lesion; however, it is limited to lesions diagnosed as cTis (intramucosal cancer)/cT1a (SM1) by endoscopic findings and judged to be amenable to en-bloc resection by appropriate endoscopic treatment method.[29] Same as with esophageal and gastric cancer, a comprehensive judgment must be made by making full use of WLI findings and the JNET classification which is an IEE-ME finding.

SUMMARY

WLI findings are still very important for detection and characterization of early neoplastic lesions in the GI tract. However, IEE-ME is becoming increasingly important and is quite useful for qualitative diagnosis of GI neoplastic lesions. Regarding the diagnosis of invasion depth and tumor extent, different diagnostic modalities should be selected depending on each organ. IEE-ME is extremely useful for diagnosis of invasion depth in ESCC and colorectal cancer, whereas macroscopic findings of

WLI are still useful in BAC and gastric cancer. IEE-ME is also useful for diagnosis of tumor extent in BAC and gastric cancer, whereas chromoendoscopy with indigo carmine is useful in colorectal cancer and iodine staining is indispensable in ESCC to recognize clear demarcation line when endoscopic resection is performed.

CLINICS CARE POINTS

- Understanding the macroscopic type according to the Paris classification.
- In ESCC, (1) WLI and IEE are used for detection of the tumor; however, iodine staining is also very easy to detect the lesion, (2) WLI and IEE-ME findings (based on the Japan Esophageal Society classification) are used to diagnose the invasion depth of the tumor, (3) iodine staining is indispensable for clear demarcation when endoscopic resection is performed.
- In BAC, (1) WLI and IEE-ME are used for detection and characterization of the tumor, and (2) WLI findings are used for diagnosis of invasion depth.
- In gastric cancer, (1) WLI is used for detection, (2) IEE-ME with MESDA-G is used for qualitative diagnosis including differentiation of the tumor; however, histology should be confirmed by targeted biopsy, (3) invasion depth is diagnosed based on WLI findings, and (4) IEE-ME is used for diagnosis of tumor extent but chromoendoscopy with indigo carmine is sometimes useful
- In colorectal cancer, (1) WLI is used for detection, (2) qualitative diagnosis and diagnosis of invasion depth are made based on WLI findings including macroscopic type classification, however, IEE-ME with the JNET classification is very useful for those diagnoses and its importance is increasing in recent years, and (3) chromoendoscopy with indigo carmine is useful for diagnosis of tumor extent, although it is often unnecessary due to clear demarcation.

FUNDING

None.

DISCLOSURE

None.

REFERENCES

1. The Paris endoscopic classification of superficial neoplastic lesions. esophagus, stomach, and colon: November 30 to December 1, 2002. Gastrointest Endosc 2003;58(6):S3–43.
2. Muto M, Minashi K, Yano T, et al. Early detection of superficial squamous cell carcinoma in the head and neck region and esophagus by narrow band imaging: a multicenter randomized controlled trial. J Clin Oncol 2010;28(9):1566–72.
3. Shimizu Y, Omori T, Yokoyama A, et al. Endoscopic diagnosis of early squamous neoplasia of the esophagus with iodine staining: high-grade intra-epithelial neoplasia turns pink within a few minutes. J Gastroenterol Hepatol 2008;23(4): 546–50.
4. Takeuchi M, Houjou Y, Kobayashi T, et al. Endoscopic diagnosis for superficial esophageal SCC. Stomach Intest (Tokyo) 2020;55(5):489–500.
5. Inoue T, Ishihara R, Shibata T, et al. Endoscopic imaging modalities for diagnosing the invasion depth of superficial esophageal squamous cell carcinoma: a systematic review. Esophagus 2022;19(3):375–83.

6. Kumagai Y, Inoue H, Nagai K, et al. Magnifying endoscopy, stereoscopic micro-scopy, and the microvascular architecture of superficial esophageal carcinoma. Endoscopy 2002;34(5):369–75.

7. Oyama T, Inoue H, Arima M, et al. Prediction of the invasion depth of superficial squamous cell carcinoma based on microvessel morphology: magnifying endo-scopic classification of the Japan Esophageal Society. Esophagus 2017;14(2): 105–12.

8. Kitagawa Y, Ishihara R, Ishikawa H, et al. Esophageal cancer practice guidelines 2022 edited by the Japan esophageal society: part 1. Esophagus 2023;20(3): 343–72.

9. The Japan Esophagus Society. Japanese classification of esophageal cancer, The. 12th Edition. Tokyo: Kanehara & Co. Ltd; 2022.

10. Shaheen NJ, Falk GY, Iyer PG, et al. ACG Clinical Guideline: Diagnosis and Man-agement of Barrett's Esophagus. Am J Gastroenterol 2016;111(1):30–50.

11. Sharma P, Dent J, Armstrong D, et al. The development and validation of an endoscopic grading system for Barrett's esophagus: the Prague C & M criteria. Gastroenterology 2006;131(5):1392–9.

12. Thonsani N, Abu Dayyeh BK, Sharma P, et al. ASGE Technology Committee sys-tematic review and meta-analysis assessing the ASGE Preservation and Incorpo-ration of Valuable Endoscopic Innovations thresholds for adopting real-time imaging-assisted endoscopic targeted biopsy during endoscopic surveillance of Barrett's esophagus. Gastrointest Endosc 2016;83(4):684–98.

13. Muto M, Yao K, Kaise M, et al. Magnifying endoscopy simple diagnostic algorithm for early gastric cancer (MESDA-G). Dig Endosc 2016;28(4):379–93.

14. Goda K, Fujisaki J, Ishihara R, et al. Newly developed magnifying endoscopic classification of the Japan Esophageal Society to identify superficial Barrett's esophagus-related neoplasms. Esophagus 2018;15(3):153–9.

15. May A, Günter E, Roth F, et al. Accuracy of staging in early oesophageal cancer using high resolution endoscopy and high resolution endosonography: a compar-ative, prospective, and blinded trial. Gut 2004;53(5):634–40.

16. Chemaly M, Scalone O, Durivage G, et al. Miniprobe EUS in the pretherapeutic assessment of early esophageal neoplasia. Endoscopy 2008;40(1):2–6.

17. Ishihara R, Arima M, Iizuka T, et al. Endoscopic submucosal dissection/endo-scopic mucosal resection guidelines for esophageal cancer. Dig Endosc 2020; 32(4):452–93.

18. Nakayoshi T, Tajiri H, Matsuda K, et al. Magnifying endoscopy combined with nar-row band imaging system for early gastric cancer: correlation of vascular pattern with histopathology (including video). Endoscopy 2004;36(12):1080–4.

19. Nawada Y, Hirasawa D, Matsuda T, et al. Endoscopic diagnosis for gastric can-cer associated with Helicobacter pylori. Stomach Intest (Tokyo) 2020;55(5): 557–71.

20. Tsuji Y, Kato M, Inoue T, et al. Integrated diagnostic strategy for the invasion depth of early gastric cancer by conventional endoscopy and EUS. Gastrointest Endosc 2015;82(3):452–9.

21. Tsuji Y, Hayashi Y, Ishihara R, et al. Diagnostic value of endoscopic ultrasonogra-phy for the depth of gastric cancer suspected of submucosal invasion: a multi-center prospective study. Surg Endosc 2023;37(4):3018–28.

22. Yao K, Anagnostopoulos GK, Ragunath K. Magnifying endoscopy for diagnosing and delineating early gastric cancer. Endoscopy 2009;41(5):462–7.

23. Japanese Gastric Cancer Association. Japanese Gastric Cancer Treatment Guidelines 2021 (6th edition). Gastric Cancer 2023;26(1):1–25.

24. Matsuda T, Kawano H, Chiu HM. Screening colonoscopy: What is the most reliable modality for the detection and characterization of colorectal lesions? Dig Endosc 2015;27(Suppl. 1):25–9.
25. Douglas AC, Christopher DJ, Amy RM, et al. Adenoma Detection Rate and Risk of Colorectal Cancer and Death. N Engl J Med 2014;370(14):1298–306.
26. Vogelstein B, Fearon ER, Hamilton SR, et al. Genetic alterations during colorectal-tumor development. N Engl J Med 1988;319(9):525–32.
27. Kuramoto S, Oohara T. Minute cancers arising de novo in the human large intestine. Cancer 1988;61(4):829–34.
28. Sawyer SJ, Cerar A, Hanby AM, et al. Molecular characteristics of serrated adenomas of the colorectum. Gut 2002;51(2):200–6.
29. Japanese Society for. the Cancer of the Colon and Rectum. JSCCR guidelines 2022 for the treatment of colorectal cancer. Kanehara & Co. Ltd, Tokyo; 2022.
30. Kudo S, Lambert R, Alle JI, et al. Nonpolypoid neoplastic lesions of the colorectal mucosa. Gastrointest Endosc 2008;68(4 Suppl):S3–47.
31. Saito Y, Obara T, Watari J, et al. Invasion depth diagnosis of depressed type early colorectal cancers by combined use of videoendoscopy and chromoendoscopy. Gastrointest Endosc 1998;48(4):362–70.
32. Kudo S, Hirota S, Nakajima T, et al. Colorectal tumours and pit pattern. J Clin Pathol 1994;47(10):880–5.
33. Health Canada. Health Canada warns Canadians of potential cancer risk associated with gentian violet. Available at: https://healthycanadians.gc.ca/recall-alert-rappel-avis/hc-sc/2019/70179a-eng.php. Accessed June 12, 2019.
34. Hamamoto N, Hirata I, Yasumoto S, et al. Diagnosis of the Depth of Invasion by Endoscopic Ultrasonography in Early Colorectal Carcinomas. Stomach Intest (Tokyo) 2004;39(10):1375–86.
35. Sano Y, Tanaka S, Kudo S, et al. Narrow-band imaging (NBI) magnifying endoscopic classification of colorectal tumors proposed by the Japan NBI Expert Team. Dig Endosc 2016;28(5):526–33.

Endoscopic Diagnosis of Extra-Luminal Cancers

Ross C.D. Buerlein, MD*, Vanessa M. Shami, MD

KEYWORDS

- Endoscopic ultrasound • Cytology • Fine needle aspiration • Fine needle biopsy
- Staging

KEY POINTS

- Endoscopic ultrasound (EUS) offers the opportunity to identify, stage, and sample lesions in many different locations outside of the gastrointestinal lumen including the pancreatico-biliary system.
- EUS can be used to identify, sample, and stage posterior mediastinal lesions and lung cancers adjacent to the esophagus.
- EUS allows for sampling of masses in the peritoneum, which otherwise may require laparoscopy to access.
- In cholangiocarcinoma, there is an increased risk of seeding the EUS needle tract, so EUS-directed tissue acquisition should be avoided in potential transplant candidates.
- Cholangiocarcinoma is often challenging to acquire adequate tissue for diagnosis, so multimodality sampling via endoscopic retrograde cholangiopancreatography (ERCP) is generally recommended.

INTRODUCTION

Traditionally utilized only for gastrointestinal (GI) lumen pathologies, endoscopy has emerged as a powerful tool in diagnosing various malignancies outside of the GI lumen, allowing for minimally invasive and accurate staging and tissue acquisition (TA) of numerous organ systems. This rapidly evolving field has had a bourgeoning of significant advancements in high-definition endoscopic visualization, virtual chromoendoscopy, endoscopic ultrasound (EUS)-guided TA, multi-modality sampling, novel DNA markers, contrast-enhanced (CE) EUS, and artificial intelligence (AI), which continue to push the boundaries of diagnostic capabilities. This comprehensive review highlights the latest breakthroughs in the endoscopic diagnosis of extraluminal malignancies, shedding light on the expanding horizons of precision medicine and its potential to transform cancer care.

Division of Gastroenterology and Hepatology, University of Virginia Health System, Box 800708, Charlottesville, VA 22908, USA
* Corresponding author.
E-mail address: RCB9N@uvahealth.org

Gastrointest Endoscopy Clin N Am 34 (2024) 19–36
https://doi.org/10.1016/j.giec.2023.07.001
1052-5157/24/© 2023 Elsevier Inc. All rights reserved.

DISCUSSION
Pancreatic Cancer

Pancreatic ductal adenocarcinoma represents up to 95% of all pancreatic cancers and is currently the fourth leading cause of cancer-related death in the United States. The incidence of pancreatic cancer is increasing, and by 2030 it is predicted to become the second leading cause of cancer-related death.[1–4] Survival rate is determined by the stage at diagnosis and surgical resectability. Unfortunately, at least 80% of pancreatic cancers are considered advanced stage, and more than half have systemic metastases at initial diagnosis.[4–6] Accurate staging and TA for proper histologic assessment are critical in determining a treatment strategy.

Diagnostic modalities

EUS is generally considered the most sensitive imaging modality for detecting pancreatic cancers of any type, particularly small lesions, and it also allows for TA. The sensitivity of EUS for detecting pancreatic cancer ranges from 89% to 100%, with an accuracy of 94% to 96%[7] and provides for the assessment of

- Lesion size
- Lesion location within the pancreas
- Vascular involvement
- Lymphadenopathy
- Metastatic disease

However, cross-sectional imaging is considered the most accurate for staging and determining surgical resectability.[4,7] The sensitivity for detecting pancreatic cancer with a pancreatic-protocol computed tomographic (CT) scan ranges from 76% to 96% and typically provides a better assessment of vascular involvement than MRI (**Fig. 1**A, B).[1]

Contrast-enhanced endoscopic ultrasound

EUS is relatively operator-dependent, and detecting small lesions and differentiating chronic pancreatitis changes from a pancreatic adenocarcinoma can be challenging. In recent years, the advent of CE EUS, which uses a microbubble-based contrast agent to enhance visualization, has been shown to improve the diagnostic abilities of EUS[4].

- A study[8] of 101 patients with pancreatic lesions underwent EUS followed by CE EUS and showed a diagnostic yield of 64% with standard EUS compared with 91% with CE EUS (odds ratio 7.8, 95% confidence interval [CI] 2.7–30.2).
- A meta-analysis of 2644 patients using CE EUS to diagnose pancreatic adenocarcinoma found a pooled sensitivity of 90% and specificity of 89%.[9]

Endoscopic ultrasound with real-time elastography

EUS with real-time elastography (RTE) measures tissue density by assessing distortion after a predetermined pressure is applied to the tissue.[4] This technology is highly operator-dependent, and its clinical utility has yet to be fully elucidated regarding the assessment of solid pancreatic masses. A study of 50 consecutive patients with pancreatic masses who had previously undergone nondiagnostic EUS-fine needle aspiration (FNA) subsequently underwent CE EUS and EUS RTE. The study demonstrated high levels of accuracy (84%) for both techniques.[10]

Nuances of endoscopic ultrasound in pancreatic cancer

When performing EUS of pancreatic cancer, the endoscopist should note multiple characteristics of the mass:

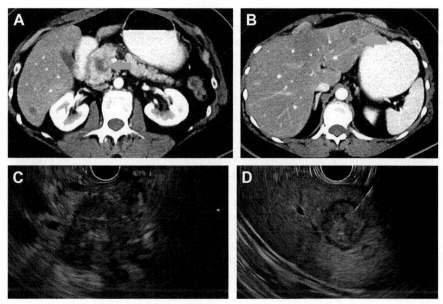

Fig. 1. (*A, B*) A 60 year old woman presenting with painless jaundice. Laboratory assessment revealed normal liver enzymes and a normal CA-19-9 level of 9 (U/mL). CT showed a 4 cm mass in the head of the pancreas which is noted by the (*green arrow, A*) and a 1 cm rim-enhancing hypoechoic density in the left lobe of the liver which is noted by the (*green arrow, B*). (*C*) The same patient underwent EUS-FNA of the liver lesion was consistent with a metastatic deposit of pancreatic adenocarcinoma. Note that the lesion is hypoechoic with poorly defined borders. (*D*) Endoscopic ultrasound-guided FNA of a liver lesion confirmed to be a metastatic deposit of pancreatic adenocarcinoma.

- Size (maximal dimension)
- Location within the pancreas
- Echodensity of the lesion
- Borders (poorly or well-defined)
- Presence of any cystic components within the mass
- Ductal dilation upstream from the mass
- Relationship with major vessels

Care should also be taken to assess for and document the following:

- Any visible lymph nodes for features of metastatic disease, which typically include size ≥ 1 cm, well-defined borders, rounded shape, and/or appearing hypoechoic.
- Left and right lobes of the liver for any evidence of metastatic deposits, which may appear as hypoechoic, hyperechoic, or even isoechoic lesions[7] (**Fig. 1C, D**).
- The presence of ascites.
- The presence of extra-pancreatic lesions, and, when identified, EUS-directed sampling of these areas should be performed first, as tissue confirmation of malignancy at any of these distant sites is confirmatory for advanced-stage disease.[7] If negative, the primary pancreatic mass should be sampled.

Fine needle aspiration versus biopsy
EUS-guided TA can be performed using FNA or fine needle biopsy (FNB) with needles of various sizes and shapes. FNA is generally considered the reference standard for EUS

TA, but it has significant limitations in its ability to retain cellular architecture and stroma, thus leading to the advent of the FNB needle.[11] The overall efficacy of FNB compared with FNA differs between studies. A meta-analysis[12] of 11 trials, including 833 patients with solid pancreatic masses, compared the performance characteristics of using 22-gauge FNA versus FNB needles and showed (for cases of pancreatic cancer) comparable diagnostic accuracy (relative risk [RR] 1.02, 95% CI 0.97–1.08) and pooled sensitivities of 90.4% (86.3%–94.5%) with FNA and 93.1% (87.9%–98.5%) with FNB ($P = .46$). Additionally, FNB had a nonsignificant trend for requiring fewer needle passages to obtain pathologic confirmation (-0.32, $P = .07$) compared with FNA.[12] However, the location of the mass and the angle of approach for the pathway of the needle from the transducer to the mass impact needle selection. For example, FNA needles (compared with FNB needles) are typically considered more flexible and may be better suited for lesions requiring significant scope or elevator angulation.[13] A study[14] of 32 patients with solid pancreatic lesions undergoing EUS TA were randomized to undergo FNA or FNB (all using 22-gauge needles), resulting in FNA having significantly higher diagnostic accuracy on the first pass (FNA 93.8% vs FNB 28.1%, $P < .001$) which was partially explained by 5 cases having technical failure due to the inability to advance the FNB needle into the target tissue, though the samples obtained via FNA had more contamination compared with those by FNB ($P = .036$).

FNB needles are manufactured in numerous different shapes.[15] The most common is the

- Franseen needle, which has 3 cutting edges.
- Fork-tip needle, which has 2 cutting surfaces opposite each other.
- Reversed bevel needle, which has a side hole along the needle length with a cutting surface facing the opposite direction.

Ex vivo studies[15] have shown different rates of resistance against needle advancement based on different needle manufacturers and shapes. A network meta-analysis[16] of 16 randomized-control trials with 1934 patients showed Franseen needles and fork-tip needles both out-performed reversed bevel needles and FNA needles for accuracy and there were no differences between any of the needles (various FNB shapes and FNA needles) when rapid on-site evaluation (ROSE) was used. Therefore, needle selection (FNA vs FNB, needle gauge, FNB tip shape) is up to the discretion and preference of the endoscopist and should be tailored to the following:

- Position of the lesion
- Angulation of the echoendoscope
- Degree of elevator usage required to access the lesion

Number of needle passages during sampling

The number of optimal needle passages into a lesion during EUS TA is debated, though there are data to support that more than 4 needle passages do not increase the diagnostic yield.

- A multicenter prospective study[17] assessing the number of EUS-FNA needle passages necessary to reach a histologic diagnosis in 202 patients with pancreatic malignancies showed 4 passages detected malignancy with 93% sensitivity for masses ≥ 2 cm; however, for masses ≤ 2 cm in size, 6 passages detected malignancy with 82% sensitivity, indicating that smaller lesions may require more passages for adequate TA.
- A study[18] of 61 patients with solid pancreatic masses undergoing EUS-FNA showed the diagnosis was obtained on the first passage in 62% of cases, on

the second passage in 15%, on the third passage in 15%, and on the fourth passage in only 3%, indicating that more than 3 passages are likely of little clinical utility.

Endoscopic ultrasound tissue acquisition techniques

There must be a clear consensus on the most optimal EUS TA technique. Most experts agree on performing the "fanning" technique in which different areas of the lesion are sampled during the back-and-forth motion of the needle during a single needle passage.[4] Once the needle is positioned inside a lesion, the stylet is advanced to the end of the needle to push out any tissue obtained from the track of the needle passage. Following this, several different techniques can be applied:

- *Slow-pull technique*: The stylet is slowly withdrawn from the length of the needle throughout the sampling process, creating a slight suction force that pulls tissue into the needle.
- *Suction technique*: The stylet is removed, and a syringe is attached to the needle hub, followed by the application of negative pressure throughout the sampling process. A dry suction technique uses a syringe of air, whereas a wet suction technique involves pre-flushing the needle with water or heparin before suction.

A prospective study[19] of 92 cases of solid pancreatic cancers assessed the diagnostic yield of EUS FNA using the slow-pull and standard suction (SS) techniques and showed the SS group had higher rates of blood contamination (2.19 vs 1.50, $P < .001$) and lower rates of diagnostic samples (30.0% vs 41.8%, $P = .003$) but no differences in the diagnostic yield, sensitivity, specificity, or cellularity of samples between the groups. A meta-analysis[20] of 6 studies including 418 patients compared wet versus dry suction and demonstrated more optimal performance characteristics with wet suction compared with dry suction (pooled odds of sample adequacy was 3.18 [95% CI 1.82–5.54, $P = .001$]) with comparable rates of blood contamination and histologic accuracy.

Complications of endoscopic ultrasound-directed sampling of pancreatic lesions

EUS TA is considered generally safe with low complication rates, including

- Bleeding: 1% to 4%
- Pancreatitis: 1% to 2%,
- Perforation: less than 0.5%.[21]

These risks may be increased when sampling smaller lesions and pancreatic neuroendocrine tumors.[4,22]

Rapid on-site evaluation

The necessity of ROSE with tissue sampling in pancreatic cancer has been debated. In a multicenter (14 centers in 8 countries) randomized prospective noninferiority study[23] of 800 patients with solid pancreatic lesions assessed the diagnostic accuracy of EUS-FNB with and without ROSE and found comparable results (96.4% with ROSE vs 97.4% without ROSE, $P = .396$).

Endoscopic ultrasound-directed portal vein sampling

The entire GI system has venous drainage via the portal circulation. EUS-directed portal vein (EUS-PV) sampling has detected tumor cells of various GI origin that otherwise may not be present in systemic circulation due to hepatic filtration.[24] In cases of pancreatic cancer, EUS-PV has detected circulating tumor cells (CTCs) at higher rates than matched peripheral blood samples, and these CTCs can be used for drug sensitivity analysis, molecular testing, and even clinical prognostication.[25] For example, in a single center study of 18 patients with pancreaticobiliary cancers, blood obtained via EUS-PV contained CTCs in all 18 cases, whereas CTCs were found in the peripheral blood of only 4 cases.[26] Although the clinical utility of EUS-PV is still being determined and not being used routinely, it serves as a potential future diagnostic modality.

Gallbladder Cancer

Diagnosing gallbladder cancer can prove challenging and is influenced by the size of the mass, the location of the tumor within the gallbladder, the shape of the gallbladder itself, and the proximity of the mass to other neighboring structures (namely the liver and the biliary tree). EUS can help assess this, though visualization of the entire gallbladder may be limited by the shape and location of the gallbladder in relation to the gastric and duodenal anatomy (**Fig. 2**). Therefore, imaging (cross-sectional and trans-abdominal ultrasound) should be performed separately from EUS during the workup of possible gallbladder cancer.[27,28] Malignancy can arise within a gallbladder polyp and often follows a similar sequence of adenoma-to-cancer as colorectal polyps,[29] and multiple surgical societal guidelines recommend consideration for cholecystectomy with gallbladder polyps greater than 10 mm in size.[30,31]

Role of endoscopic ultrasound in gallbladder cancer
EUS is not required to diagnose gallbladder cancer. However, it can play an essential role in

- Determining the depth of invasion/staging
- TA
- Assessment for metastatic spread to regional lymph nodes or the liver

EUS is not necessary for staging alone; however, Lee and colleagues[32] assessed the diagnostic accuracy of high-resolution transabdominal ultrasound and EUS in cases of gallbladder cancer and showed that the 2 modalities are similar (sensitivity 82.7% and 86.2%, respectively).

Endoscopic ultrasound-directed tissue acquisition
EUS-FNA for TA in cases of the gallbladder can be helpful but is not indicated. Singla and colleagues[33] assessed the performance characteristics of EUS-FNA in 98

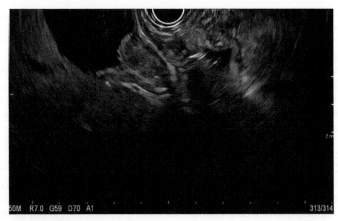

Fig. 2. EUS of a gallbladder mass.

patients with gallbladder cancer resulting in biliary obstruction and showed a sensitivity of 90.81% and a specificity and accuracy of 100%.

Although complication rates from EUS-FNA of a gallbladder mass are low, important variables must be considered before proceeding. Owing to the risk of bile leakage and associated biliary peritonitis and acute cholecystitis, puncture into the lumen of the gallbladder is not recommended. There is also a small risk of dissemination of malignant cells into the needle tract or peritoneum.[28,33]

Endoscopic retrograde cholangiopancreatography-directed sampling

Endoscopic retrograde cholangiography (ERC) with brushings or biopsies for gallbladder cancer is generally considered significantly lower than EUS-FNA. Hijioka and colleagues[34] assessed 83 patients with gallbladder cancer who underwent EUS-FNA (n = 31) or ERC (n = 53) and showed that the diagnostic sensitivity of EUS-FNA was significantly higher than ERC (96% vs 47.4%, respectively, $P<$ .001). Therefore, except in rare circumstances, ERC is not recommended as the initial test for TA in cases of suspected gallbladder cancer.

Cholangiocarcinoma

Cholangiocarcinoma (CCA) is a malignancy arising from biliary epithelial cells anywhere in the biliary tree and is divided into subtypes based on location:

- Intra-hepatic
- Hilar
- Distal

Endoscopic diagnostic capabilities and overall treatment vary depending on the location and size of the tumor. These malignancies are desmoplastic and typically present as biliary strictures, though mass-like lesions are seen (particularly for intrahepatic lesions).[35]

Diagnostic modalities

Obtaining effective TA for diagnosis is notoriously challenging in CCA. ERC allows for cytologic assessment from brushings, histologic assessment from forceps biopsies, cellular acquisition for fluorescent in-situ hybridization (FISH), and genetic testing. ERC remains the reference standard for nonsurgical diagnostic TA in CCA (**Fig. 3**). Some unique features of CCA can make TA challenging and limited. For example, accessing intrahepatic CCA may be difficult via ERC, tight strictures may limit the ability of a device to traverse that segment, lesions with a high degree of fibrosis or desmoplasia can limit the cellularity of samples, and some lesions have submucosal (rather than mucosal) spread. Therefore, multimodality sampling is highly recommended.[36]

Endoscopic retrograde cholangiography-directed biliary brushings and biopsies

Brush cytology is widely considered the initial test of choice due to its ease, high specificity, and safety. However, brush cytology sensitivity is low, with studies ranging from 6% to 75%, though most agree the sensitivity averages in the 30% to 50% range.[36,37] Pediatric and standard biopsy forceps can be passed through the duodenoscope working channel and into the biliary tree under fluoroscopic guidance, and most studies suggest the sensitivity of this ranges from 40% to 88%.[36] The addition of biopsies to brushings improves diagnostic yield. A meta-analysis[38] of 730 patients with indeterminate biliary strictures showed the pooled sensitivity to be 45% with brushings alone, 48% with biopsies alone, and 59% with the combination of both modalities.

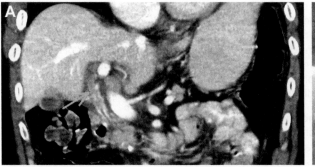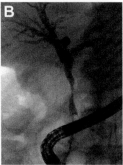

Fig. 3. (*A, B*) A 58 year old man presenting with progressively worsening jaundice without pain but with low-grade fevers. Laboratory assessment showed AST 677 U/L, ALT 1045 U/L, alkaline phosphatase 898 U/L, and total bilirubin 4.8 mg/dL. CT (*A*) revealed increased wall enhancement of the proximal common bile duct (as noted by the *green arrow*) with intra-hepatic ductal dilation. Subsequent ERC-directed cholangiogram (*B*) confirmed a stricture of the proximal common bile duct, which was brushed with cytology, confirming a ductal adenocarcinoma, consistent with cholangiocarcinoma.

Cholangioscopy

Single-operated cholangioscopy allows for direct visualization of the biliary epithelium and targeted biopsies. Certain visualized features of strictures are indicative of a malignancy:[39]

- Irregularly dilated and tortuous vessels
- Friability
- Nodularity
- Papillary changes

Some cholangioscopy platforms allow for the usage of narrow-band imaging, which has been shown to further highlight these features.[40] Additionally, applying AI using a convolutional neural network to cholangioscopy may improve the diagnostic accuracy for CCA. For example, Njei[41] et al. performed a systemic review of 4 studies, including 934 patients undergoing cholangioscopy for CCA, and found an accuracy of 94.9%, a sensitivity of 94.7%, and a specificity of 92.1%.

Fluorescence in situ hybridization

FISH targets specific chromosomal alterations associated with CCA, and the addition of it to brush cytology and/or biopsy forceps significantly increases the diagnostic sensitivity. In a retrospective study, Baroud and colleagues[42] assessed trimodality sampling (brush cytology, forceps biopsies, and FISH) in 204 patients, including 104 with malignancy, and showed the sensitivity for diagnosing malignancy to be

- 17.3% with brush cytology alone
- 40.4% with brush cytology + forceps biopsy
- 58.7% with brush cytology + FISH
- 68.3 with combining brushings + forceps biopsies + FISH (*P*< .001 for all comparisons)

Next-generation sequencing

Next-generation sequencing (NGS) allows for detecting oncogenic mutations in specific genes of interest and adding NGS to brush cytology samples can significantly improve the sensitivity for diagnosing CCA.[43] In the future, the array of mutations associated with CCA is expected to increase, leading to a further increase in the sensitivity of this diagnostic modality for CCA.

Endoscopic ultrasound in cholangiocarcinoma

EUS can be beneficial in diagnosing CCA and, in many studies, is superior to ERC-directed sampling.[44] For example, in a meta-analysis[45] of 294 patients with malignant biliary strictures, the sensitivity of a tissue diagnosis of malignancy with ERCP (including brushings and biopsy forceps) was 49% but with EUS was 75%. However, as occurred in this study, many studies include distal biliary strictures related to pancreatic cancer as an etiology of malignant biliary strictures, which will falsely lower the diagnostic abilities of ERC. As with other malignancies, EUS allows for assessment and sampling of the primary lesion of interest and regional lymph nodes or the presence of metastatic disease. EUS-FNA in cases of CCA comes with a much higher risk of needle tract seeding than in other malignancies and is generally considered an absolute contraindication in patients who are potential liver transplantation candidates or if the sample can be obtained via alternative methods.[46] However, the data on this are mixed:

- Heimbach and colleagues[47] assessed 191 patients with locally advanced (unresectable) perihilar CCA and showed that 83% of the 16 patients who underwent FNA of the primary tumor (13 percutaneous and 3 EUS-FNA) had peritoneal metastases at the time of operative staging compared with only 8% of those who did not undergo FNA ($P = .0097$).
- A study[48] of 150 patients with confirmed CCA, 61 of whom underwent EUS-FNA, showed that EUS-directed sampling had no impact on overall or progression-free survival.

Lung cancer

Accurate lung cancer diagnosis and staging are essential to guide patients to appropriate surgical or systemic therapy in non-small cell lung cancer. T4 and/or N2-3 and/or M1-disease is considered nonsurgical.

Diagnosis of lung cancer

Primary centrally located lung cancers adjacent to the esophagus are accessible by EUS and more straightforward to approach than with CT-guided techniques. Most of the time, cross-sectional imaging reveals a mass adjacent to the esophagus, and EUS and tissue sampling are recommended (**Fig. 4**). The sensitivity for EUS-directed sampling ranges from 88% to 100%.[49–52]

Staging of lung cancer

EUS also has a role in staging lung cancer by assessing for tumor invasion (T4 disease), defined as the invasion in the mediastinum, centrally located large vessels, or vertebrae. A retrospective study evaluated 308 patients with T4 cancer, and EUS had sensitivity, specificity, and positive and negative predictive values of 88%, 98%, 70%, and 99%, respectively.[53] Additionally, EUS can evaluate for malignant pleural effusion. Mediastinoscopy is an invasive and somewhat morbid technique to assess lymph node involvement in patients with lung cancer. EUS combined with endobronchial ultrasound (EBUS) is less invasive and less expensive.[54–60] Using EUS in this setting reduces the need for surgery and cost.[61,62]

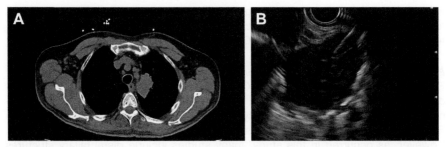

Fig. 4. (*A, B*) A 73 year old woman who presented with persistent dry cough underwent CT chest (*A*) showing a left lung mass which was located near the esophagus. EUS (*B*) confirmed the mass and EUS-FNA was performed.

EUS access stations	EBUS access stations
2L (left high paratracheal)	- 2R
4L (left low paratracheal)	- 3P
7 (subcarinal)	- 4R
8 (para-esophageal)	- 4L
9 (pulmonary ligament)	- 7
EUS can access at times	- 10R
5	- 10L
6	- 11R
EUS also access	- 11L
Celiac axis	
Left adrenal gland	
Left liver lobe	

Combining EBUS with EUS increases the diagnostic accuracy for mediastinal staging in lung cancer.[63–70] This approach is included in the European Societies' combined guidelines of European Society of Gastrointestinal Endoscopy, the European Society of Thoracic Surgeons, and the European Respiratory Society.[71,72]

Another advantage of EUS is the ability to quickly assess and sample the left adrenal gland, the fifth leading site of metastasis for lung cancer (**Fig. 5**).[73] As the left adrenal gland is adjacent to the proximal stomach, it is easy to access and, if involved by cancer, would deem someone unresectable. EUS can also restage after chemotherapy and radiation.

Mediastinal Lesions

EUS-FNA can evaluate and sample posterior mediastinal lesions. These lesions can be malignant (including lymphoma, lung cancer, metastatic disease, gastrointestinal stromal tumor [GIST], and spindle cell tumors) or benign (including abscess, leiomyoma, and granulomatous disease). A meta-analysis of 76 studies of 9310 patients found a pooled sensitivity of 88% and specificity of 96%.[74] Many of these studies are over 15 year old, and the yield is most likely higher with newer-generation FNA and FNB needles.

Risks of EUS-sampling of posterior mediastinal lesions are low. A pooled review of prospective studies revealed a 0.43% risk of complications, including bleeding, pain, and perforation.[75] Mediastinitis rarely occurs; most cases are related to cyst sampling.

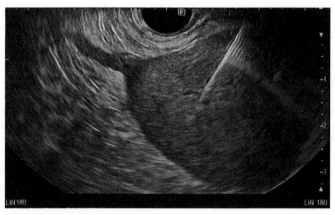

Fig. 5. EUS-FNA of a large mass seen in the left adrenal gland in a patient with suspected metastatic lung cancer (confirmed on cytology).

Liver Lesions

EUS-FNA provides access to liver lesions that may be difficult to biopsy percutaneously. EUS images the left hepatic lobe, the proximal right lobe, and the hilum. It can be used for TA for primary hepatic cancers such as hepatocellular carcinoma (HCC) or for documenting metastatic disease. EUS is particularly useful in sub-cm liver lesions, which CT or MRI often misses.

Diagnosis of focal liver lesions

Focal liver lesions can be malignant (HCC, CCA) or benign. This discussion will be limited to the malignant lesion (HCC) (**Fig. 6**). Intrahepatic CCA has already been discussed above.

In a study by Awad and colleagues, in all 14 patients with HCC and metastatic lesions who underwent both dynamic CT and EUS, EUS identified liver lesions of 0.3 to 14 cm in size.[76] Additionally, EUS identified new lesions less than 0.5 cm in 28% of the patients. In a prospective single-center study evaluating 17 patients who

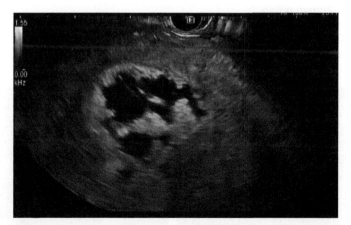

Fig. 6. EUS image of a hepatocellular carcinoma in the liver of a 78 year old man with cirrhosis.

underwent cross-sectional imaging and EUS, 9 had liver tumors. EUS-FNA established a tissue diagnosis in 8 of 9 cases. The diagnostic accuracy of transabdominal US, CT, MRI, and EUS-FNA were 38%, 69%, 92%, and 94%, respectively.[77]

Diagnosis of metastatic disease to the liver

EUS staging of esophageal, gastric, pancreatic, biliary, and lung cancers should include liver inspection for metastases (**Fig. 7**). Identification of metastatic disease often has treatment and prognostic implications. In Okasha and colleagues[78] study, 730 patients underwent prospective EUS staging of various cancers, including 575 of pancreaticobiliary origin. All patients additionally underwent CT or MRI. EUS detected liver metastases in 118 patients (16.2%), while CT or MRI detected metastasis in 82 (11.2%). EUS missed metastases in 6 patients, while CT and MRI missed metastases in 42 patients. Therefore, inspecting the liver during EUS must be performed routinely when staging luminal and extraluminal cancers.

Contrast harmonic-endoscopic ultrasound for diagnosis of liver lesions

Recently, contrast agents such as sonazoid and lumason have been used to help identify lesions in the liver. In a study by Minaga and colleagues,[79] CH-EUS was superior in accuracy to B-mode EUS and multidetector CT for detecting left lobe metastases. Another small trial of 30 consecutive patients showed similar results.[80] The Asian Federation of Societies for Ultrasound in Medicine and Biology recommends that CH-EUS be used to characterize and guide EUS-FNA only in liver lesions with unclear margins or in the case of previous negative EUS-FNA.[81]

Peritoneal masses

Sampling peritoneal masses for diagnosis or to document distant disease is essential for prognosis and therapy. Additionally, advances in personalized cancer treatments make histology even more critical. Laparoscopy is the gold standard but invasive. Paracentesis is easy and safe but has a low sensitivity for diagnosis.[82] EUS-FNA of peritoneal lesions and metastases has a good safety profile and is quite sensitive in diagnosing malignant lesions.[83] With FNB needles, EUS-FNB can obtain enough tissue for IHC staining in peritoneal lesions. A prospective series[84] showed 63.6% sensitivity, 100% specificity, and 66.7% accuracy of EUS-FNB of peritoneal lesions. Adequate tissue for IHC stain was found in 25 of 30 passes (80%).

Cancer of unknown origin

Many cancers of unknown origins are adenocarcinomas. Most originate from the pancreas, GI lumen, female reproductive tract, or lung. PET scan helps evaluate the entire body; however, this is unrevealing in some patients.

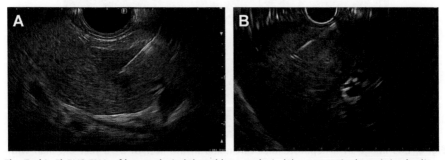

Fig. 7. (A, B) EUS-FNA of hypoechoic (A) and hyperechoic (B) metastatic deposit in the liver.

Esophagogastroduodenoscopy (EGD) plays a role in assessing the GI lumen, and EUS-FNA allows for TA of lymph nodes, peritoneum, or other extraluminal organs in hopes that cytologic analysis will be able to identify the cancer origin.[85] Additionally, if there is a suspicion that the source is pancreaticobiliary (presence of elevated CA-19–9 or cytology),[86] EUS is superior to cross-sectional imaging in identifying small lesions.

SUMMARY

Technological advancements in endoscopy over the last several decades have allowed for endoscopic staging and minimally invasive TA of malignancies outside of the lumen of the GI tract, supplanting previously conventional diagnostic modalities. As new technologies and advancements emerge, the diagnostic capabilities of endoscopy in this field will continue to grow.

CLINICS CARE POINTS

- EUS is the most sensitive modality for imaging the pancreas. It offers the least-invasive approach for accurate TA, while cross-sectional imaging is generally still preferred to determine surgical resection.
- Although EUS offers the ability for TA and can assist in staging gallbladder cancers, its usage is generally not required.
- Multimodality sampling via ERC (brushings, biopsies, FISH) is generally recommended in CCAs due to this malignancy's fibrotic and desmoplastic nature. EUS-TA can be helpful in diagnostic confirmation, but this comes with a risk of seeding the needle tract and peritoneum and is not recommended in potential transplant candidates.
- EUS can be used to identify, sample, and stage posterior mediastinal lesions and lung cancers adjacent to the esophagus.
- EUS allows for sampling of masses in the peritoneum, which otherwise may require laparoscopy to access.

DISCLOSURE

V.M. Shami: Consultant for Olympus America, Cook Medical, and Boston Scientific. R.C.D. Buerlein: Nothing to disclose.

REFERENCES

1. Wood LD, Canto MI, Jaffee EM, et al. Pancreatic Cancer: Pathogenesis, Screening, Diagnosis, and Treatment. Gastroenterology 2022;163(2):386–402.e1.
2. Rahib L, Smith BD, Aizenberg R, et al. Projecting cancer incidence and deaths to 2030: the unexpected burden of thyroid, liver, and pancreas cancers in the United States. Cancer Res 2014;74(11):2913–21.
3. Hussain A, Weimer DS, Mani N. Diagnosing Pancreatic Adenocarcinoma With Contrast-Enhanced Ultrasonography: A Literature Review of Research in Europe and Asia. Cureus 2022;14(2):e22080.
4. Salom F, Prat F. Current role of endoscopic ultrasound in the diagnosis and management of pancreatic cancer. World J Gastrointest Endosc 2022;14(1):35–48.
5. Siegel RL, Miller KD, Fuchs HE, et al. Cancer Statistics, 2021. CA Cancer J Clin 2021;71(1):7–33.

6. Bockhorn M, Uzunoglu FG, Adham M, et al. Borderline resectable pancreatic cancer: a consensus statement by the International Study Group of Pancreatic Surgery (ISGPS). Surgery 2014;155(6):977–88.

7. Young Bang TR. *Endosonography*. Vol 4. Endoscopic ultrasound and pancreatic tumors. Amsterdam, The Netherlands: Elsevier; 2019.

8. Buxbaum J, Ko C, Varghese N, et al. Qualitative and Quantitative Contrast-enhanced Endoscopic Ultrasound Improves Evaluation of Focal Pancreatic Lesions. Clin Gastroenterol Hepatol 2020;18(4):917–25.e4.

9. Lin LZ, Li F, Liu Y, et al. Contrast-Enhanced Ultrasound for differential diagnosis of pancreatic mass lesions: a meta-analysis. Med Ultrason 2016;18(2):163–9.

10. Iordache S, Costache MI, Popescu CF, et al. Clinical impact of EUS elastography followed by contrast-enhanced EUS in patients with focal pancreatic masses and negative EUS-guided FNA. Med Ultrason 2016;18(1):18–24.

11. James TW, Baron TH. A comprehensive review of endoscopic ultrasound core biopsy needles. Expert Rev Med Devices 2018;15(2):127–35.

12. Facciorusso A, Bajwa HS, Menon K, et al. Comparison between 22G aspiration and 22G biopsy needles for EUS-guided sampling of pancreatic lesions: A meta-analysis. Endosc Ultrasound 2020;9(3):167–74.

13. Matsubayashi H, Matsui T, Yabuuchi Y, et al. Endoscopic ultrasonography guided-fine needle aspiration for the diagnosis of solid pancreaticobiliary lesions: Clinical aspects to improve the diagnosis. World J Gastroenterol 2016;22(2): 628–40.

14. Strand DS, Jeffus SK, Sauer BG, et al. EUS-guided 22-gauge fine-needle aspiration versus core biopsy needle in the evaluation of solid pancreatic neoplasms. Diagn Cytopathol 2014;42(9):751–8.

15. Matsunami Y, Itoi T, Tsuchiya T, et al. Objective evaluation of the resistance forces of 22-gauge EUS-FNA and fine-needle biopsy needles. Endosc Ultrasound 2023; 12(2):251–8.

16. Gkolfakis P, Crinò SF, Tziatzios G, et al. Comparative diagnostic performance of end-cutting fine-needle biopsy needles for EUS tissue sampling of solid pancreatic masses: a network meta-analysis. Gastrointest Endosc 2022;95(6): 1067–77.e15.

17. Mohamadnejad M, Mullady D, Early DS, et al. Increasing Number of Passes Beyond 4 Does Not Increase Sensitivity of Detection of Pancreatic Malignancy by Endoscopic Ultrasound-Guided Fine-Needle Aspiration. Clin Gastroenterol Hepatol 2017;15(7):1071–8.e2.

18. Teodorescu C, Gheorghiu M, Zaharie T, et al. Endoscopic ultrasonography-fine needle aspiration of solid pancreatic masses: Do we need the fourth pass? A prospective study. Diagn Cytopathol 2021;49(3):395–403.

19. Bor R, Vasas B, Fábián A, et al. Prospective comparison of slow-pull and standard suction techniques of endoscopic ultrasound-guided fine needle aspiration in the diagnosis of solid pancreatic cancer. BMC Gastroenterol 2019;19(1):6.

20. Ramai D, Singh J, Kani T, et al. Wet- versus dry-suction techniques for EUS-FNA of solid lesions: A systematic review and meta-analysis. Endosc Ultrasound 2021; 10(5):319–24.

21. Gonzalo-Marin J, Vila JJ, Perez-Miranda M. Role of endoscopic ultrasound in the diagnosis of pancreatic cancer. World J Gastrointest Oncol 2014;6(9):360–8.

22. Katanuma A, Maguchi H, Yane K, et al. Factors predictive of adverse events associated with endoscopic ultrasound-guided fine needle aspiration of pancreatic solid lesions. Dig Dis Sci 2013;58(7):2093–9.

23. Crinò SF, Di Mitri R, Nguyen NQ, et al. Endoscopic Ultrasound-guided Fine-needle Biopsy With or Without Rapid On-site Evaluation for Diagnosis of Solid Pancreatic Lesions: A Randomized Controlled Non-Inferiority Trial. Gastroenterology 2021;161(3):899–909.e5.

24. Ryou M, DeWitt JM, Das KK, et al. AGA Clinical Practice Update on Interventional EUS for Vascular Investigation and Therapy: Commentary. Clin Gastroenterol Hepatol 2023. https://doi.org/10.1016/j.cgh.2023.03.027.

25. Chapman CG, Waxman I. EUS-Guided Portal Venous Sampling of Circulating Tumor Cells. Curr Gastroenterol Rep 2019;21(12):68.

26. Catenacci DV, Chapman CG, Xu P, et al. Acquisition of Portal Venous Circulating Tumor Cells From Patients With Pancreaticobiliary Cancers by Endoscopic Ultrasound. Gastroenterology 2015;149(7):1794–803.e4.

27. Al-Haddad M. Endosonographic ultrasound in bile duct, gallbladder, and ampullary lesions. In: Robert H, Hawes PF, Varadarajulu S, editors. Endosonography. Amsterdam, The Netherlands: Elsevier; 2019. p. 201–25.

28. Hijioka S, Nagashio Y, Ohba A, et al. The Role of EUS and EUS-FNA in Differentiating Benign and Malignant Gallbladder Lesions. Diagnostics 2021;11(9). https://doi.org/10.3390/diagnostics11091586.

29. Choi TW, Kim JH, Park SJ, et al. Risk stratification of gallbladder polyps larger than 10 mm using high-resolution ultrasonography and texture analysis. Eur Radiol 2018;28(1):196–205.

30. Wennmacker SZ, Lamberts MP, Di Martino M, et al. Transabdominal ultrasound and endoscopic ultrasound for diagnosis of gallbladder polyps. Cochrane Database Syst Rev 2018;8(8):Cd012233.

31. Foley KG, Lahaye MJ, Thoeni RF, et al. Management and follow-up of gallbladder polyps: updated joint guidelines between the ESGAR, EAES, EFISDS and ESGE. Eur Radiol 2022;32(5):3358–68.

32. Lee JS, Kim JH, Kim YJ, et al. Diagnostic accuracy of transabdominal high-resolution US for staging gallbladder cancer and differential diagnosis of neoplastic polyps compared with EUS. Eur Radiol 2017;27(7):3097–103.

33. Singla V, Agarwal R, Anikhindi SA, et al. Role of EUS-FNA for gallbladder mass lesions with biliary obstruction: a large single-center experience. Endosc Int Open 2019;7(11):E1403–9.

34. Hijioka S, Hara K, Mizuno N, et al. Diagnostic yield of endoscopic retrograde cholangiography and of EUS-guided fine needle aspiration sampling in gallbladder carcinomas. J Hepatobiliary Pancreat Sci 2012;19(6):650–5.

35. Coronel M, Lee JH, Coronel E. Endoscopic Ultrasound for the Diagnosis and Staging of Biliary Malignancy. Clin Liver Dis 2022;26(1):115–25.

36. Elmunzer BJ, Maranki JL, Gómez V, et al. ACG Clinical Guideline: Diagnosis and Management of Biliary Strictures. Am J Gastroenterol 2023;118(3):405–26.

37. Buckholz AP, Brown RS Jr. Cholangiocarcinoma: Diagnosis and Management. Clin Liver Dis 2020;24(3):421–36.

38. Navaneethan U, Njei B, Lourdusamy V, et al. Comparative effectiveness of biliary brush cytology and intraductal biopsy for detection of malignant biliary strictures: a systematic review and meta-analysis. Gastrointest Endosc 2015;81(1):168–76.

39. Parsa N, Khashab MA. The Role of Peroral Cholangioscopy in Evaluating Indeterminate Biliary Strictures. Clin Endosc 2019;52(6):556–64.

40. Shin IS, Moon JH, Lee YN, et al. Efficacy of narrow-band imaging during peroral cholangioscopy for predicting malignancy of indeterminate biliary strictures (with videos). Gastrointest Endosc 2022;96(3):512–21.

41. Njei B, McCarty TR, Mohan BP, et al. Artificial intelligence in endoscopic imaging for detection of malignant biliary strictures and cholangiocarcinoma: a systematic review. Ann Gastroenterol 2023;36(2):223–30.

42. Baroud S, Sahakian AJ, Sawas T, et al. Impact of trimodality sampling on detection of malignant biliary strictures compared with patients with primary sclerosing cholangitis. Gastrointest Endosc 2022;95(5):884–92.

43. Kamp E, Dinjens WNM, van Velthuysen MF, et al. Next-generation sequencing mutation analysis on biliary brush cytology for differentiation of benign and malignant strictures in primary sclerosing cholangitis. Gastrointest Endosc 2023;97(3): 456–65.e6.

44. Orzan RI, Pojoga C, Agoston R, et al. Endoscopic Ultrasound in the Diagnosis of Extrahepatic Cholangiocarcinoma: What Do We Know in 2023? Diagnostics 2023; 13(6). https://doi.org/10.3390/diagnostics13061023.

45. De Moura DTH, Moura EGH, Bernardo WM, et al. Endoscopic retrograde cholangiopancreatography versus endoscopic ultrasound for tissue diagnosis of malignant biliary stricture: Systematic review and meta-analysis. Endosc Ultrasound 2018;7(1):10–9.

46. Gleeson FC, Lee JH, Dewitt JM. Tumor Seeding Associated With Selected Gastrointestinal Endoscopic Interventions. Clin Gastroenterol Hepatol 2018; 16(9):1385–8.

47. Heimbach JK, Sanchez W, Rosen CB, et al. Trans-peritoneal fine needle aspiration biopsy of hilar cholangiocarcinoma is associated with disease dissemination. HPB (Oxford) 2011;13(5):356–60.

48. El Chafic AH, Dewitt J, Leblanc JK, et al. Impact of preoperative endoscopic ultrasound-guided fine needle aspiration on postoperative recurrence and survival in cholangiocarcinoma patients. Endoscopy 2013;45(11):883–9.

49. Vazquez-Sequeiros E, Levy MJ, Van Domselaar M, et al. Diagnostic yield and safety of endoscopic ultrasound-guided fine needle aspiration of central mediastinal lung masses. Diagn Ther Endosc 2013;2013:150492.

50. Varadarajulu S, Hoffman BJ, Hawes RH, et al. EUS-guided FNA of lung masses adjacent to or abutting the esophagus after unrevealing CT-guided biopsy or bronchoscopy. Gastrointest Endosc 2004;60(2):293–7.

51. Annema JT, Veseliç M, Rabe KF. EUS-guided FNA of centrally located lung tumours following a non-diagnostic bronchoscopy. Lung Cancer 2005;48(3): 357–61 [discussion: 363-4].

52. Hernandez A, Kahaleh M, Olazagasti J, et al. EUS-FNA as the initial diagnostic modality in centrally located primary lung cancers. J Clin Gastroenterol 2007; 41(7):657–60.

53. Varadarajulu S, Schmulewitz N, Wildi SM, et al. Accuracy of EUS in staging of T4 lung cancer. Gastrointest Endosc 2004;59(3):345–8.

54. Pedersen BH, Vilmann P, Folke K, et al. Endoscopic ultrasonography and real-time guided fine-needle aspiration biopsy of solid lesions of the mediastinum suspected of malignancy. Chest 1996;110(2):539–44.

55. Verma A, Jeon K, Koh WJ, et al. Endobronchial ultrasound-guided transbronchial needle aspiration for the diagnosis of central lung parenchymal lesions. Yonsei Med J 2013;54(3):672–8.

56. Silvestri GA, Hoffman BJ, Bhutani MS, et al. Endoscopic ultrasound with fine-needle aspiration in the diagnosis and staging of lung cancer. Ann Thorac Surg 1996;61(5):1441–5 [discussion: 1445-6].

57. Vilmann P, Annema J, Clementsen P. Endosonography in bronchopulmonary disease. Best Pract Res Clin Gastroenterol 2009;23(5):711–28.

58. Annema JT, van Meerbeeck JP, Rintoul RC, et al. Mediastinoscopy vs. endoso- nography for mediastinal nodal staging of lung cancer: a randomized trial. JAMA 2010;304(20):2245–52.

59. Wiersema MJ, Vilmann P, Giovannini M, et al. Endosonography-guided fine- needle aspiration biopsy: diagnostic accuracy and complication assessment. Gastroenterology 1997;112(4):1087–95.

60. Herth FJ, Eberhardt R, Vilmann P, et al. Real-time endobronchial ultrasound guided transbronchial needle aspiration for sampling mediastinal lymph nodes. Thorax 2006;61(9):795–8.

61. Rintoul RC, Glover MJ, Jackson C, et al. Cost effectiveness of endosonography versus surgical staging in potentially resectable lung cancer: a health economics analysis of the ASTER trial from a European perspective. Thorax 2014;69(7): 679–81.

62. Sharples LD, Jackson C, Wheaton E, et al. Clinical effectiveness and cost- effectiveness of endobronchial and endoscopic ultrasound relative to surgical staging in potentially resectable lung cancer: results from the ASTER randomised controlled trial. Health Technol Assess 2012;16(18):1–75, iii-iv.

63. Zhang R, Ying K, Shi L, et al. Combined endobronchial and endoscopic ultrasound-guided fine needle aspiration for mediastinal lymph node staging of lung cancer: a meta-analysis. Eur J Cancer 2013;49(8):1860–7.

64. Korevaar DA, Crombag LM, Cohen JF, et al. Added value of combined endobron- chial and oesophageal endosonography for mediastinal nodal staging in lung cancer: a systematic review and meta-analysis. Lancet Respir Med 2016;4(12): 960–8.

65. Vilmann P, Krasnik M, Larsen SS, et al. Transesophageal endoscopic ultrasound- guided fine-needle aspiration (EUS-FNA) and endobronchial ultrasound-guided transbronchial needle aspiration (EBUS-TBNA) biopsy: a combined approach in the evaluation of mediastinal lesions. Endoscopy 2005;37(9):833–9.

66. Wallace MB, Pascual JM, Raimondo M, et al. Minimally invasive endoscopic stag- ing of suspected lung cancer. JAMA 2008;299(5):540–6.

67. Herth FJ, Krasnik M, Kahn N, et al. Combined endoscopic-endobronchial ultra- sound-guided fine-needle aspiration of mediastinal lymph nodes through a single bronchoscope in 150 patients with suspected lung cancer. Chest 2010;138(4): 790–4.

68. Szlubowski A, Zieliński M, Soja J, et al. A combined approach of endobronchial and endoscopic ultrasound-guided needle aspiration in the radiologically normal mediastinum in non-small-cell lung cancer staging–a prospective trial. Eur J Car- dio Thorac Surg 2010;37(5):1175–9.

69. Liberman M, Sampalis J, Duranceau A, et al. Endosonographic mediastinal lymph node staging of lung cancer. Chest 2014;146(2):389–97.

70. Oki M, Saka H, Ando M, et al. Endoscopic ultrasound-guided fine needle aspira- tion and endobronchial ultrasound-guided transbronchial needle aspiration: Are two better than one in mediastinal staging of non-small cell lung cancer? J Thorac Cardiovasc Surg 2014;148(4):1169–77.

71. Vilmann P, Clementsen PF, Colella S, et al. Combined endobronchial and esoph- ageal endosonography for the diagnosis and staging of lung cancer: European Society of Gastrointestinal Endoscopy (ESGE) Guideline, in cooperation with the European Respiratory Society (ERS) and the European Society of Thoracic Surgeons (ESTS). Endoscopy 2015;47(6):c1.

72. Vilmann P, Clementsen PF, Colella S, et al. Combined endobronchial and esoph- ageal endosonography for the diagnosis and staging of lung cancer: European

Society of Gastrointestinal Endoscopy (ESGE) Guideline, in cooperation with the European Respiratory Society (ERS) and the European Society of Thoracic Surgeons (ESTS). Endoscopy 2015;47(6):545–59.

73. Riihimäki M, Hemminki A, Fallah M, et al. Metastatic sites and survival in lung cancer. Lung Cancer 2014;86(1):78–84.

74. Puli SR, Batapati Krishna Reddy J, Bechtold ML, et al. Endoscopic ultrasound: it's accuracy in evaluating mediastinal lymphadenopathy? A meta-analysis and systematic review. World J Gastroenterol 2008;14(19):3028–37.

75. Wang KX, Ben QW, Jin ZD, et al. Assessment of morbidity and mortality associated with EUS-guided FNA: a systematic review. Gastrointest Endosc 2011;73(2): 283–90.

76. Awad SS, Fagan S, Abudayyeh S, et al. Preoperative evaluation of hepatic lesions for the staging of hepatocellular and metastatic liver carcinoma using endoscopic ultrasonography. Am J Surg 2002;184(6):601–4 [discussion: 604-5].

77. Singh P, Erickson RA, Mukhopadhyay P, et al. EUS for detection of the hepatocellular carcinoma: results of a prospective study. Gastrointest Endosc 2007;66(2): 265–73.

78. Okasha HH, Wifi MN, Awad A, et al. Role of EUS in detection of liver metastasis not seen by computed tomography or magnetic resonance imaging during staging of pancreatic, gastrointestinal, and thoracic malignancies. Endosc Ultrasound 2021;10(5):344–54.

79. Minaga K, Kitano M, Nakai A, et al. Improved detection of liver metastasis using Kupffer-phase imaging in contrast-enhanced harmonic EUS in patients with pancreatic cancer (with video). Gastrointest Endosc 2021;93(2):433–41.

80. Oh D, Seo DW, Hong SM, et al. The usefulness of contrast-enhanced harmonic EUS-guided fine-needle aspiration for evaluation of hepatic lesions (with video). Gastrointest Endosc 2018;88(3):495–501.

81. Kitano M, Yamashita Y, Kamata K, et al. The Asian Federation of Societies for Ultrasound in Medicine and Biology (AFSUMB) Guidelines for Contrast-Enhanced Endoscopic Ultrasound. Ultrasound Med Biol 2021;47(6):1433–47.

82. Allen VA, Takashima Y, Nayak S, et al. Assessment of False-negative Ascites Cytology in Epithelial Ovarian Carcinoma: A Study of 313 Patients. Am J Clin Oncol 2017;40(2):175–7.

83. DeWitt J, LeBlanc J, McHenry L, et al. Endoscopic ultrasound-guided fine-needle aspiration of ascites. Clin Gastroenterol Hepatol 2007;5(5):609–15.

84. Kongkam P, Orprayoon T, Yooprasert S, et al. Endoscopic ultrasound guided fine needle biopsy (EUS-FNB) from peritoneal lesions: a prospective cohort pilot study. BMC Gastroenterol 2021;21(1):400.

85. Breslin NP, Wallace MB. EUS: a role in metastatic cancer with undiagnosed primary? Gastrointest Endosc 2001;54(6):793–6.

86. Krishna SG, Rao BB, Ugbarugba E, et al. Diagnostic performance of endoscopic ultrasound for detection of pancreatic malignancy following an indeterminate multidetector CT scan: a systemic review and meta-analysis. Surg Endosc 2017;31(11):4558–67.

Endoscopic Ultrasound in Cancer Staging

Harry R. Aslanian, MD*, Thiruvengadam Muniraj, MD,
Anil Nagar, MD, David Parsons, MD

KEYWORDS

- Endoscopic ultrasound • Cancer staging • Esophageal adenocarcinoma
- Gastric cancer • Cholangiocarcinoma • Pancreatic adenocarcinoma
- Colorectal cancer

KEY POINTS

- Endoscopic ultrasound (EUS) is superior to CT, MRI, or PET for N staging, and the addition of FNA improves diagnostic accuracy.
- EUS is superior to CT, MRI, or PET for T staging but less sensitive in distinguishing T1a from T1b lesions.
- MDCT is the gold standard for vascular staging; however, EUS may provide complimentary information, with a high negative predictive value for involvement of the spleno-portal confluence.
- EUS is less accurate in restaging after chemoradiation due to inflammation and fibrosis from tumor.
- EUS in combination with endoscopic assessment remains the preferred method of locoregional staging, providing complementary information to cross-sectional imaging.

Accurate staging of cancer is crucial for prognosis and treatment planning. Cross-sectional imaging with CT, MRI, and PET scans provides important assessments for metastatic disease and prominent lymphadenopathy. Endoscopic ultrasound (EUS) is an important tool to improve the accuracy of locoregional staging.

Effective utilization of EUS for accurate tumor staging can reduce superfluous surgical procedures, reducing the cost of cancer care and improving morbidity and mortality.[1] The most widely used tumor classification is the American Joint Committee on Cancer Tumor, Node, Metastasis (TNM) classification. This system classifies the tumor based on the depth of tumor invasion (T), degree of lymph node involvement (N), and presence or absence of metastasis (M). EUS is the gold standard for

Department of Medicine, Section Digestive Diseases, Yale University School of Medicine, New Haven, CT, USA
* Corresponding author. Department of Internal Medicine, Section Digestive Diseases, Yale University School of Medicine, 333 Cedar Street, New Haven, CT 06520.
E-mail address: Harry.Aslanian@Yale.edu

Gastrointest Endoscopy Clin N Am 34 (2024) 37–49
https://doi.org/10.1016/j.giec.2023.09.009
1052-5157/24/© 2023 Elsevier Inc. All rights reserved.
giendo.theclinics.com

determining tumor depth and lymph node involvement (T- and N-stage) and provides direct tissue or nodal sampling.[2,3]

A careful endoscopic examination before EUS helps to identify the anatomic location and extent of the tumor and if any additional luminal disease is present. Overall, EUS plays a vital role that aids in guiding therapy through collaboration between gastroenterologists and oncologists.

ESOPHAGEAL CANCER

Esophageal adenocarcinoma (EAC) is the most common esophageal malignancy in the United States, with a higher incidence in Caucasian males. Risk factors include obesity, smoking, gastro-esophageal reflux disease (GERD), and Barrett's esophagus.[4] In contrast, esophageal squamous cell carcinoma is more common worldwide, with a higher incidence in Blacks and risk factors including smoking, alcohol, achalasia, radiation, human papillomavirus (HPV), and caustic ingestion. Preoperative EUS staging for EAC is associated with a 42.1% reduction in mortality.[5] Superficial tumors (Tumor in situ [Tis] which does not extend beyond the basement membrane or T1s which does not extend beyond the lamina propria) are amenable to curative endoscopic resection, whereas T1b (submucosal involvement) may require esophagectomy but can also be considered for endoscopic mucosal resection (EMR) or endoscopic submucosal dissection (ESD) with low-risk features. EUS can evaluate lymphadenopathy and tumor depth before endoscopic resection. Patients with T1b tumors without lymphadenopathy have good outcomes after endoscopic resection.[5,6] T1b tumors have lymph node involvement up to 16%[7] and may require esophagectomy. However, due to the morbidity of esophagectomy, the American Gastroenterology Association states that EMR or ESD can be considered for T1b tumors with low-risk features (good to moderate differentiation, no lymphatic involvement, and <500 μm invasion into submucosa). T2 or T3 tumors warrant esophagectomy regardless of nodal involvement, and patients with nodal involvement or advanced tumors (T2–T4) require chemoradiotherapy with subsequent restaging.

Studies showed that EUS accuracy in T and N staging in EAC is superior to MRI, CT, or PET staging.[7–9] A meta-analysis showed EUS sensitivity from 81.6% to 92.4% for T staging,[10] compared with CT scan, with sensitivity of 42% to 60%.[8,11] Recent improvements in cross-sectional imaging, however, have narrowed the gap, and prior studies may underestimate the sensitivity of current imaging. Other studies have identified lower accuracy of EUS staging of superficial esophageal malignancy with a 2010 meta-analysis finding EUS and pathologic T staging concordance of only 65% for superficial EAC.[12] Retrospective comparisons of EUS to pathologic staging found inaccurate EUS staging in approximately one-fifth of early-stage disease.[13] In indeterminate cases, histologic staging is more accurate than EUS staging, and endoscopic resection or limited EMR may be pursued.

Assessment of the nodal stage is crucial in TNM staging. The presence of pathologic lymph nodes warrants adding chemoradiation in T2 disease, where node-negative cancers are treated with surgery alone. Nodes to assess include cervical, periesophageal, carinal, and perigastric nodes. Celiac lymphadenopathy indicates poor prognosis. Suspicious features of lymph nodes are size greater than 1 cm, round, hypoechoic, and sharply demarcated. When all four criteria are met, there is an 85% chance of malignancy.[14] EUS accuracy for nodal staging varies (59.5%–100%),[15] but adding fine needle aspiration (FNA) to EUS greatly increases the diagnostic accuracy (90%–99.4%).[10,16,17] Peritumoral nodes are typically not sampled to avoid false positive results and tumor spread to nodes. EUS/FNA has greater sensitivity than CT for nodal involvement and is less expensive than CT-guided lymph node biopsy.[18]

EUS staging of bulky tumors is limited by the size of the echoendoscope (12 mm), which is larger than traditional (10 mm) gastroscopes. Passing the EUS scope in EAC with high-grade stricture is difficult and risky. Pre-dilation may help, and dilation up to 16 mm is safe, but dilation beyond 18 mm increases perforation rate.[19,20] EUS miniprobe through the working channel or thin caliber endobronchial ultrasound (EBUS) scope may be used for staging, but their accuracy is inferior to the EUS scope.[19–21] EUS staging may not be necessary in obstructing tumors as failure to pass a gastroscope through a malignant stricture indicates locally advanced disease (T3).[22] EUS staging after chemoradiation is harder due to the difficulty of differentiating fibrosis, necrosis, and inflammation.[23]

For early EAC, EUS and endoscopic visualization are used to assess submucosal involvement. EMR or ESD may remove lesions limited to the mucosa without lymphadenopathy or metastasis, providing histologic staging and resection adequacy determination (**Fig. 1**).

GASTRIC CANCER

Gastric cancer is the fifth most common cancer and the third leading cause of cancer death worldwide and fourth most common gastrointestinal (GI) malignancy in the United States.[24] Risk factors include smoking, obesity, high sodium and nitrate-containing diet, *Helicobacter pylori*, Epstein-Barr virus (EBV) infection, Menetrier's disease, and prior gastric surgery.[4] Like EAC, accurate staging is imperative in determining the treatment course. Early gastric cancer without nodal involvement may be treated with endoscopic resection, whereas stage 1B or higher cancers benefit from perioperative or adjuvant chemotherapy. Advanced metastatic disease receives sequential chemotherapy, but prognosis is poor with less than 1-year median survival.[24] Favorable prognostic factors include well-differentiated carcinoma, size less than 2 cm, cancer limited to the mucosa, and absence of lymph node involvement.[25]

CT, MRI, and PET-CT are important staging modalities but less accurate for T and N staging.[26] EUS is more accurate and sensitive for locoregional staging with sensitivities of 85% for distinguishing T1 from T2 disease and 87% for T1a from T1b disease. EUS reliably distinguishes between early and advanced tumors with a sensitivity of 86% and a specificity of 90%.

EUS nodal staging has variable results due to limited visualization. Meta-analyses report sensitivities from 16.7% to 95.3% and specificities from 48.4% to 100%. A later meta-analysis showed 83% sensitivity and 67% specificity.[27,28] EUS and multi-

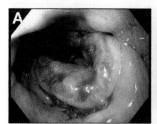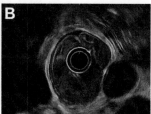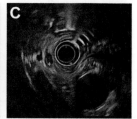

Fig. 1. Upper endoscopy revealed an ulcerated mass at the GE junction (*A*). Endoscopic Ultrasound showed invasion through the muscularis propria (*B*). Two lymph nodes were identified (*C*). The lesion was staged as T3N1.

detector computed tomography (MDCT) have complementary roles in staging gastric cancer, and additional liver evaluation during EUS improves overall accuracy.[29]

EUS identifies the wall layers from which the lesion originates and characterizes gastric subepithelial tumors, with FNA/B providing tissue for diagnosis. Fine needle aspiration/biopsy (FNA/B) can distinguish between a leiomyoma and gastrointestinal stromal tumor (GIST), using c-kit and Dog-1 immunohistochemistry, and mitotic counts classify the malignant behavior.[30–32] EUS accuracy for GISTs ranges from 71% to 100%.[32,33] GISTs are classified based on size, echo pattern, margins, and mitotic rate, with high-risk tumors requiring resection and adjuvant imatinib therapy.

EUS is valuable in diagnosing and staging gastric lymphoma. The depth of involvement is crucial to determine treatment, with mucosa-limited mucosa-associated lymphoid tissue (MALT) lymphoma potentially responding to *H pylori* eradication, whereas advanced MALT lymphoma and diffuse B-cell lymphoma require chemotherapy, radiation, or surgery.[34] EUS is also used to confirm treatment response and detect early recurrence.[35]

EUS limitations for gastric cancer diagnosis include difficulty identifying distal nodal metastasis, reduced accuracy in differentiating T1a and T1b lesions and overstaging of tumors greater than 3 cm, and poorly differentiated tumors[35] (**Fig. 2**).

PANCREATIC CANCER

Pancreatic cancer carries the highest mortality of all malignancies and is the third leading cause of cancer death in the United States.[36] Pancreatic cancer frequently presents at a late stage, with 80% to 90% of patients presenting with nonoperable or metastatic disease.[37] Surgery is the only curative treatment of pancreatic cancer, and negative margins at surgery increase the 5-year survival rate to 40%.[38] EUS has a sensitivity of 99% for diagnosis, superior to CT (55%), and detects more peripancreatic, subcarinal, and peri-celiac lymph nodes and local vascular invasion.[39] Multidetector high-resolution CT (MDHCT) and MRI have reduced the imaging superiority of EUS, but EUS remains key in detecting lesions less than 2 cm.[40–42] EUS has advantages over CT in T staging, vascular invasion of spleno-portal confluence, and N staging as shown in a meta-analysis.[43] Furthermore, EUS has been shown to be reliable in ruling out pancreatic cancer, with a negative predictive value of approximately 100%.[44]

EUS allows for obtaining tissue through FNA or FNB, which can confirm a pancreatic cancer diagnosis and differentiate from other malignancies and benign disorders, including autoimmune pancreatitis or mass forming chronic pancreatitis.[44,45] The

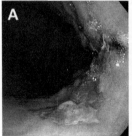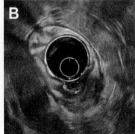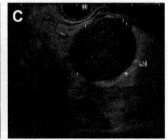

Fig. 2. Upper endoscopy shows a gastric mass (*A*) in the antrum. EUS shows the lesion arising from the mucosal layer and invading the muscularis propria (*B*). The serosa was intact and the adjacent liver was uninvolved. At least five peritumoral nodes were seen, including a 2.5 × 2.3 cm gastrohepatic node (*C*). The lesion was staged as T3N2.

addition of FNA/B to obtain histopathology increases the overall accuracy; however, the sensitivity is reduced in patients with chronic pancreatitis (73.9% compared with 91.3% in patients without chronic pancreatitis).[46] FNB needles may provide greater diagnostic accuracy with fewer needle passes required and may increase the yield for molecular testing of tumor samples.[47] On-site pathology is helpful in increasing the diagnostic yield of EUS-FNA; however, it may not be needed when using FNB needles.[48]

EUS/FNA complications are rare (0%–2.5%), including hemorrhage, perforation, infection, and acute pancreatitis. EUS-FNA/B is the "gold standard" for the tissue diagnosis of pancreatic cancer. EUS allows for lesion identification, staging, acquiring tissue for diagnosis, and performing therapeutic interventions such as celiac neurolysis for pain relief, EUS-guided fiducial or brachytherapy seed placement, direct injection of chemotherapy agents or tumor ablation, and EUS-guided biliary drainage.[49]

EUS is crucial for monitoring pancreatic cysts, especially those with high-risk features like thick walls, thick septations, mural nodules, the presence of a mass, size greater than 3 cm, and main pancreas duct dilation.[50] EUS-FNA cyst fluid samples may be evaluated for cytology, viscosity, amylase, and carcinoembryonic antigen (CEA).[51]

Pancreatic neuroendocrine tumors (PNETs) account for 2% to 3% of pancreatic tumors, but their incidence is increasing.[52] EUS can detect PNETs as small as 2 to 5 mm, with higher sensitivity (91.7%) than CT (63.3%). CT misses a significant percentage of PNETs ≤1 to 2 cm.[53,54] EUS has a sensitivity of 87.2% and a specificity of 98% for PNET diagnosis.[55] Additional techniques aiding in diagnosis include the use of contrast-enhanced EUS to evaluate the hemodynamics and vascularity in real time, as well as FNA/FNB, which can add tissue for histologic diagnosis.[52]

EUS may have limitations in detecting and diagnosing pancreatic cancer, chronic pancreatitis, diffusely infiltrating pancreatic carcinoma, acute pancreatitis, and obstructing lesions.[56] If clinical suspicion remains high despite a negative EUS (FNA), repeat CT and/or EUS in 2 to 3 months is recommended. When there is biliary or pancreas duct obstruction, ERCP (± cholangioscopy) with intraductal sampling should be performed. EUS/FNA/B can be performed concurrently with ERCP, and positive onsite sampling can eliminate the need for intraductal sampling during ERCP and may aid in the decision to use a biliary self-expanding metal stent to alleviate biliary obstruction (**Fig. 3**).

CHOLANGIOCARCINOMA

Cholangiocarcinoma (CCA) is the most common biliary malignancy that often presents with jaundice due to intrahepatic or extrahepatic strictures.[57] Diagnosis can be difficult, as strictures without an associated mass are common.[58] Methods of diagnosis include ERCP (± cholangioscopy) with brushing and biopsy, which has a relatively low diagnostic yield in comparison to EUS/FNA of solid pancreas masses.[59] EUS with FNA is complementary to ERCP and may be effective in cases where ERCP

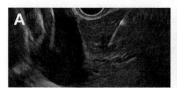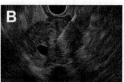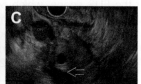

Fig. 3. EUS with FNA of a primary pancreatic mass (*A*) and liver metastasis (*B*). EUS images show a dilated bile duct with sludge and loss of plane between the mass and portal vein/superior mesenteric vein (*C*).

demonstrated negative cytology. A meta-analysis of six studies found EUS-FNA to have sensitivity of 66% and a negative likelihood ratio of 0.34.[58] Diagnostic yield of EUS was higher in patients with a mass lesion (80% sensitivity, 0.2 negative likelihood ratio). In a separate analysis comparing ERCP with brush cytology, ERCP with biopsy, ERCP with biopsy and brush cytology, or EUS with FNA showed a sensitivity of 56% for brushing, 67% for biopsy, 70.7% for brushing and biopsy, and 73.6% for EUS with FNA. There was no significant difference between EUS-FNA and brushing with biopsy.[60] EUS provides improved visualization of mass lesions and adjacent nodes, offering N staging.[61]

EUS with FNA has limitations in CCA diagnosis, especially without a mass, where the diagnostic yield is likely similar or inferior to ERCP-guided sampling. EUS also carries a risk of tumor seeding, particularly in intrahepatic CCA and liver transplant candidates and may preclude them from a potentially curative transplant. Patients with primary sclerosing cholangitis and those with biliary stents present at the time of evaluation may also have decreased diagnostic accuracy.

COLORECTAL CANCER
Rectal Cancer

Although EUS is used for lesions throughout the upper GI tract, its utility in lower GI tumors has been concentrated in staging rectal cancers. Accurate staging is important for determining the prognosis and treatment plan. EUS has an accuracy of 70% to 95% for T staging.[62] EUS is superior to cross-sectional imaging in T and N staging of rectal cancers.[62] Stage 1 lesions include T1 and T2 tumors. T1 lesions limited to the mucosa can be treated by EMR or ESD, whereas T2 lesions require surgery.[63] Locally advanced lesions (T3 or T4) or cancers with lymph node involvement (any T stage) require neoadjuvant chemoradiation to improve recurrence-free survival.[64] Careful endoscopic inspection should also be performed to assess for signs of submucosal involvement. A 2004 meta-analysis showed that EUS was superior for the detection of invasion of perirectal tissue and nodal involvement.[65] The investigators concluded that EUS was the most accurate modality and was useful in determining therapeutic strategies.

EUS for N staging in rectal cancer has varied accuracy between 63% and 85%, with a sensitivity of 76%.[66,67] Malignant nodes are typically round or ovoid, hypoechogenic and at least 5 mm on the short axis.[67] N staging presents challenges for all imaging modalities due to difficulties in distinguishing between malignant and inflammatory nodes.[68] EUS-FNA was shown to improve diagnostic yield with a sensitivity of 89%, specificity of 79%, and positive predictive value of 89%. The negative predictive value, however, was only 79%, demonstrating that false negative biopsies may occur.[69] Adding FNA to staging was shown to change treatment plans in 19% of patients.[70]

Limitations in EUS for rectal cancer include lower accuracy for N stage and difficulty differentiating invasive tumors from the hypoechoic appearance of fibrosis.[66] Other potential challenges include obstructing tumors or strictures that prevent passage of the EUS scope, which occurs in 14% of cases.[71] These cases can be handled with utilization of the EUS miniprobe. A meta-analysis of EUS miniprobe for staging of 642 cases of colon or rectal cancers found a pooled sensitivity and specificity of 91% and 98% for T1 tumors, 78% and 94% for T2 tumors, 97% and 90% for T3 or T4 tumors, and 63% and 82% for nodal staging.[72]

Colon Cancer

EUS is used less often for the diagnosis and staging of colon cancer due to the size, cumbersome nature, and frequently oblique endoscopic visualization of the EUS

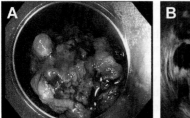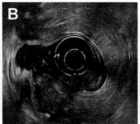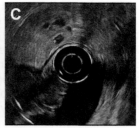

Fig. 4. Colonoscopy shows an ulcerated mass with loss of pit pattern (*A*). EUS shows submucosal involvement with thinning of the muscularis propria (*B*) and a 6-mm peritumoral node (*C*) consistent with T2N1 staging.

scope, which makes travel through the colon more difficult. A meta-analysis comparing EUS staging to histopathology showed a sensitivity and specificity of 90% and 98% for T1 lesions, 67% and 96% for T2 lesions, and 97% and 83% for T3 or T4 lesions with 59% sensitivity and 78% specificity for nodal disease.[73] The EUS miniprobe has enabled endoscopists to use a catheter-based EUS probe through a standard colonoscope. A 2017 study found staging was achieved in 39/40 patients with an accuracy of 88%. EUS miniprobe N staging was found to have an accuracy of 82% and a sensitivity of 67%.[74]

Anal Cancer

EUS accurately stages anal lesions and can help determine the proper treatment plan based on sphincter involvement. Clinical staging underestimates depth of invasion and EUS can upstage cases from T1 or T2 to T3.[75] EUS T and N stages are predictors of relapse and patient survival, whereas clinical staging was not.[76] EUS can be used again after chemoradiation to evaluate the response to therapy and choose the proper course of treatment to optimize patient survival[77] (**Fig. 4**).

NEW TECHNOLOGIES: ELASTOGRAPHY AND CONTRAST

A newer EUS modality, EUS elastography, distinguishes malignant from benign tissue by assessing the elasticity of tissues. Malignant tissues are usually harder and appear bluer on elastography imaging than benign tissue. EUS elastography outperforms EUS alone in rectal cancer staging[78] and is able to distinguish adenocarcinoma from adenomas with 94% accuracy.[79]

EUS can be performed with contrast which is called contrast harmonic EUS (CH-EUS). CH-EUS with Doppler ultrasonography allows the operator to assess the vascularity and uptake of suspected tumors and evaluate metastatic lymph nodes. CH-EUS can predict response to therapy as well as the efficacy of antiangiogenesis agents.[66] A 2013 study demonstrated 97% accuracy in differentiating benign from malignant nodes, guiding the need for FNA to avoid unnecessary cost and procedures.[80,80]

SUMMARY

In GI tumors, accurate staging is crucial to determine prognosis and treatment. CT, PET, and MRI scans are standard methods for identifying metastatic disease, but EUS has been to provide superior accuracy in locoregional staging, especially for T and N staging. FNA can also increase the accuracy of N staging and provide tissue for diagnosis. The improved accuracy of EUS over conventional imaging has reduced unnecessary surgeries and improved cost-effectiveness as well as patient outcomes. Limitations of EUS include obstructing luminal lesions, inconsistent accuracy in staging superficial tumors, and difficulty in restaging after treatment. EUS in combination with endoscopic assessment remains the preferred method of locoregional staging, providing complementary information to cross-sectional imaging. EUS is an important modality for gastroenterologists to use in collaboration with a multidisciplinary team of oncologists, radiologists, pathologists, and surgeons to improve the accuracy of tumor staging, guide therapy, and optimize patient outcomes.

CLINICS CARE POINTS

Esophageal Cancer
- When staging early esophageal cancer, incorporate the endoscopic appearance and use EMR or ESD for pathologic staging and treatment when endoscopic ultrasound (EUS) findings are indeterminate.
- When an obstructing lesion is encountered, careful dilation to 16 mm may be considered but EUS may not be needed as this is pathognomonic for T3 disease.
- In patients who receive neoadjuvant chemotherapy, EUS may be performed after treatment to determine response to therapy.

Gastric Cancer
- When encountering a stromal tumor, performing FNA/FNB may distinguish between leiomyoma and GIST and help categorize the malignant potential of GISTs and guide therapy.
- When staging H pylori-related lymphoma, EUS staging can identify patients who may respond to H pylori eradication and assess response to therapy.

Pancreatic Cancer
- When encountering a patient with pancreatic cancer, consider the potential role for EUS-guided therapeutic interventions including celiac neurolysis, fiduciary or brachytherapy seed placement, direct injection of antitumor agents, biliary drainage, and endoscopic therapy of gastric outlet obstruction.
- When evaluating patients with chronic pancreatitis, evaluate patients who may benefit from endoscopic decompression of an obstructed pancreas duct and consider that chronic pancreatitis is a risk factor for the development of pancreas cancer, which may be more difficult to detect in the setting of chronic pancreatitis.
- When performing FNA/FNB for suspected pancreatic cancer, onsite pathology can increase diagnostic yield and obviate the need for intraductal sampling during ERCP.

Cholangiocarcinoma
- When performing EUS for cholangiocarcinoma, keep in mind FNA carries a risk of tumor seeding, and intrahepatic sampling should be avoided in patients who may be transplant candidates.
- When obtaining tissue for diagnosis, remember that EUS-FNA and ERCP with brushing and biopsies have similar efficacy, and performance of both modalities may increase the diagnostic accuracy.

Colon Cancer
- When performing EUS for proximal colon cancer, use of the through–the-scope EUS miniprobe increases accessibility.
- When performing EUS for anal cancer, pay special attention to identifying sphincter involvement as this significantly impacts treatment.

DISCLOSURE

The authors have no financial or commercial interests to disclose.

REFERENCES

1. Pfau PR, Chak A. Endoscopic ultrasonography. Endoscopy 2002;34:21–8.
2. Sreenarasimhaiah J. The emerging role of endoscopic ultrasonography in cancer staging. Am J Med Sci 2005;329:247–58.
3. Amin MB, Edge S, Greene F, et al, editors. AJCC cancer staging manual. 8th edition. Springer International Publishing: American Joint Commission on Cancer; 2017.
4. Sehdev A, Catenacci DV. Gastroesophageal cancer: focus on epidemiology, classification, and staging. Discov Med 2013;16(87):103–11.
5. Harewood GC, Kumar KS. Assessment of clinical impact of endoscopic ultrasound on esophageal cancer. J Gastroenterol Hepatol 2004;19:433–9.
6. Knabe M, May A, Ell C. Endoscopic therapy in early adenocarcinomas (Barrett's cancer) of the esophagus. J Dig Dis 2015;16:363–9.
7. Endo M, Yoshino K, Kawano T, et al. Clinicopathologic analysis of lymph node metastasis in surgically resected superficial cancer of the thoracic esophagus. Dis Esophagus 2000;13:125–9.
8. Pfau PR, Perlman SB, Stanko P, et al. The role and clinical value of EUS in a multimodality esophageal carcinoma staging program with CT and positron emission tomography. Gastrointest Endosc 2007;65:377–84.
9. Takizawa K, Matsuda T, Kozu T, et al. Lymph node staging in esophageal squamous cell carcinoma: a comparative study of endoscopic ultrasonography versus computed tomography. J Gastroenterol Hepatol 2009;24:1687–91.
10. Lowe VJ, Booya F, Fletcher JG, et al. Comparison of positron emission tomography, computed tomography, and endoscopic ultrasound in the initial staging of patients with esophageal cancer. Mol Imaging Biol 2005;7:422–30.
11. Puli SR, Reddy JB, Bechtold ML, et al. Staging accuracy of esophageal cancer by endoscopic ultrasound: a meta-analysis and systematic review. World J Gastroenterol 2008;14:1479–90.
12. Young PE, Gentry AB, Acosta RD, et al. Endoscopic ultrasound does not accurately stage early adenocarcinoma or high-grade dysplasia of the esophagus. Clin Gastroenterol Hepatol 2010;8:1037–41.
13. Pouw RE, Heldoorn N, Alvarez Herrero L, et al. Do we still need EUS in the workup of patients with early esophageal neoplasia? A retrospective analysis of 131 cases. Gastrointest Endosc 2011;73:662–8.
14. Catalano MF, Sivak MV, Rice T, et al. Endosonographic features predictive of lymph node metastasis. Gastrointest Endosc 1994;40:442–6.
15. Kelly S, Harris KM, Berry E, et al. A systematic review of the staging performance of endoscopic ultrasound in gastro-oesophageal carcinoma. Gut 2001;49:534–9.
16. Chen VK, Eloubeidi MA. Endoscopic ultrasound-guided fine needle aspiration is superior to lymph node echofeatures: a prospective evaluation of mediastinal and peri-intestinal lymphadenopathy. Am J Gastroenterol 2004;99:628–33.
17. Vazquez-Sequeiros E, Wiersema MJ, Clain JE, et al. Impact of lymph node staging on therapy of esophageal carcinoma. Gastroenterology 2003;125:1626–35.
18. Harewood GC, Wiersema MJ. A cost analysis of endoscopic ultrasound in the evaluation of esophageal cancer. Am J Gastroenterol 2002;97:452–8.
19. Wallace MB, Hawes RH, Sahai AV, et al. Dilation of malignant esophageal stenosis to allow EUS guided fine-needle aspiration: safety and effect on patient management. Gastrointest Endosc 2000;51:309–13.

20. Van Dam J, Rice TW, Catalano MF, et al. High-grade malignant stricture is predictive of esophageal tumor stage. Risks of endosonographic evaluation. Cancer 1993;71:2910–7.
21. Nesje LB, Svanes K, Viste A, et al. Comparison of a linear miniature ultrasound probe and a radial-scanning echoendoscope in TN staging of esophageal cancer. Scand J Gastroenterol 2000;35:997–1002.
22. Bang JY, Ramesh J, Hasan M, et al. Endoscopic ultrasonography is not required for staging malignant esophageal strictures that preclude the passage of a diagnostic gastroscope. Dig Endosc 2016;28:650–6.
23. Isenberg G, Chak A, Canto MI, et al. Endoscopic ultrasound in restaging of esophageal cancer after neoadjuvant chemoradiation. Gastrointest Endosc 1998;48:158–63.
24. Smyth EC, Nilsson M, Grabsch HI, et al. Gastric cancer. Lancet 2020;396(10251): 635–48.
25. Kang KJ, Kim KM, Min BH, et al. Endoscopic submucosal dissection of early gastric cancer. Gut Liver 2011;5:418–26.
26. Ajani JA, D'Amico TA, Bentrem DJ, et al. Gastric cancer, version 2.2022, NCCN clinical practice guidelines in oncology. J Natl Compr Cancer Netw 2022;20(2): 167–92.
27. Kwee RM, Kwee TC. Imaging in assessing lymph node status in gastric cancer. Gastric Cancer 2009;12:6–22.
28. Mocellin S, Pasquali S. Diagnostic accuracy of endoscopic ultrasonography (EUS) for the preoperative locoregional staging of primary gastric cancer. Cochrane Database Syst Rev 2015. https://doi.org/10.1002/14651858.CD009944.
29. Ungureanu BS, Sacerdotianu VM, Turcu-Stiolica A, et al. Endoscopic ultrasound vs. computed tomography for gastric cancer staging: a network meta-analysis. Diagnostics 2021;11(1):134.
30. Papanikolaou IS, Triantafyllou K, Kourikou A, et al. Endoscopic ultrasonography for gastric submucosal lesions. World J Gastrointest Endosc 2011;3(5):86–94.
31. Caletti G, Odegaard S, Rösch T, et al. Endoscopic ultrasonography (EUS): a summary of the conclusions of the Working party for the tenth world congress of gastroenterology Los Angeles, California October, 1994. The Working Group on Endoscopic Ultrasonography. Am J Gastroenterol 1994;89:S138–43.
32. Parab TM, DeRogatis MJ, Boaz AM, et al. Gastrointestinal stromal tumors: a comprehensive review. J Gastrointest Oncol 2019;10(1):144–54, assessment. Gastroenterology. 1997;112:1087.
33. Wiersema MJ, Vilmann P, Giovannini M, et al. Endosonography-guided fine-needle aspiration biopsy: diagnostic accuracy and complication assessment. Gastroenterology 1997;112(4):1087–95.
34. Juárez-Salcedo LM, Sokol L, Chavez JC, et al. Primary gastric lymphoma, epidemiology, clinical diagnosis, and treatment. Cancer Control 2018;25(1). 1073274818778256.
35. Kim JH, Song KS, Youn YH, et al. Clinicopathologic factors influence accurate endosonographic assessment for early gastric cancer. Gastrointest Endosc 2007; 66:901–8.
36. An Update on Cancer Deaths in the United States." Centers for Disease Control and Prevention, Centers for Disease Control and Prevention, 28 Feb. 2022, Available at: https://www.cdc.gov/cancer/dcpc/research/update-on-cancer-deaths/index.htm.
37. Gonzalo-Marin J, Vila JJ, Perez-Miranda M. Role of endoscopic ultrasound in the diagnosis of pancreatic cancer. World J Gastrointest Oncol 2014;6(9):360–8.

38. Sohn TA, Yeo CJ, Cameron JL, et al. Resected adenocarcinoma of the pancreas-616 patients: results, outcomes, and prognostic indicators. J Gastrointest Surg 2000;4:567–79.
39. Kala Z, Válek V, Hlavsa J, et al. The role of CT and endoscopic ultrasound in pre-operative staging of pancreatic cancer. Eur J Radiol 2007;62:166–9.
40. Palazzo L, Roseau G, Gayet B, et al. Endoscopic ultrasonography in the diag-nosis and staging of pancreatic adenocarcinoma. Results of a prospective study with comparison to ultrasonography and CT scan. Endoscopy 1993;25:143–50.
41. Miller FH, Rini NJ, Keppke AL. MRI of adenocarcinoma of the pancreas. AJR Am J Roentgenol 2006;187:W365–74.
42. Schwarz M, Pauls S, Sokiranski R, et al. Is a preoperative multidiagnostic approach to predict surgical resectability of periampullary tumors still effective? Am J Surg 2001;182:243–9.
43. Dewitt J, Devereaux BM, Lehman GA, et al. Comparison of endoscopic ultra-sound and computed tomography for the preoperative evaluation of pancreatic cancer: a systematic review. Clin Gastroenterol Hepatol 2006;4:717–25 [quiz: 664].
44. Klapman JB, Chang KJ, Lee JG, et al. Negative predictive value of endoscopic ultrasound in a large series of patients with a clinical suspicion of pancreatic can-cer. Am J Gastroenterol 2005;100:2658–61.
45. Barthet M, Portal I, Boujaoude J, et al. Endoscopic ultrasonographic diagnosis of pancreatic cancer complicating chronic pancreatitis. Endoscopy 1996;28: 487–91.
46. Varadarajulu S, Tamhane A, Eloubeidi MA. Yield of EUS-guided FNA of pancre-atic masses in the presence or the absence of chronic pancreatitis. Gastrointest Endosc 2005;62:728–36 [quiz 751, 753].
47. van Riet PA, Erler NS, Bruno MJ, et al. Comparison of fine-needle aspiration and fine-needle biopsy devices for endoscopic ultrasound-guided sampling of solid lesions: a systemic review and meta-analysis. Endoscopy 2021;53(4):411–23.
48. Alsibai KD, Denis B, Bottlaender J, et al. Impact of cytopathologist expert on diagnosis and treatment of pancreatic lesions in current clinical practice. A series of 106 endoscopic ultrasound-guided fine needle aspirations. Cytopathology 2006;17:18–26.
49. Luz LP, Al-Haddad MA, Sey MS, et al. Applications of endoscopic ultrasound in pancreatic cancer. World J Gastroenterol 2014;20(24):7808–18.
50. Brugge WR. The role of EUS in the diagnosis of cystic lesions of the pancreas. Gastrointest Endosc 2000;52:S18–22.
51. De Angelis C, Brizzi RF, Pellicano R. Endoscopic ultrasonography for pancreatic cancer: current and future perspectives. J Gastrointest Oncol 2013;4(2):220.
52. Ishii T, Katanuma A, Toyonaga H, et al. Role of endoscopic ultrasound in the diag-nosis of pancreatic neuroendocrine neoplasms. Diagnostics 2021;11(2):316.
53. Rösch T, Lightdale CJ, Botet JF, et al. Localization of pancreatic endocrine tumors by endoscopic ultrasonography. N Engl J Med 1992;326:1721–6.
54. Khashab MA, Yong E, Lennon AM, et al. EUS is still superior to multidetector computerized tomography for detection of pancreatic neuroendocrine tumors. Gastrointest Endosc 2011;73(4):691–6.
55. Puli SR, Kalva N, Bechtold ML, et al. Diagnostic accuracy of endoscopic ultra-sound in pancreatic neuroendocrine tumors: A systematic review and meta-anal-ysis. World J. Gastroenterol. WJG 2013;19:3678.
56. Bhutani MS, Gress FG, Giovannini M, et al, No Endosonographic Detection of Tu-mor NEST Study. The No Endosonographic Detection of Tumor (NEST) Study: a

case series of pancreatic cancers missed on endoscopic ultrasonography. Endoscopy 2004;36:385–9.

57. Blechacz B, Komuta M, Roskams T, et al. Clinical diagnosis and staging of cholangiocarcinoma. Nat Rev Gastroenterol Hepatol 2011;8:512–22.

58. Navaneethan U, Njei B, Venkatesh PG, et al. Endoscopic ultrasound in the diagnosis of cholangiocarcinoma as the etiology of biliary strictures: a systematic review and meta-analysis. Gastroenterol Rep (Oxf) 2015;3(3):209–15.

59. Navaneethan U, Njei B, Venkatesh PG, et al. Fluorescence in situ hybridization for diagnosis of cholangiocarcinoma in primary sclerosing cholangitis: a systematic review and meta-analysis. Gastrointest Endosc 2014;79(943–50):e3.

60. Yoon SB, Moon SH, Ko SW, et al. Brush cytology, forceps biopsy, or endoscopic ultrasound-guided sampling for diagnosis of bile duct cancer: a meta-analysis. Dig Dis Sci 2022;67(7):3284–97.

61. Strongin A, Singh H, Eloubeidi MA, et al. Role of endoscopic ultrasonography in the evaluation of extrahepatic cholangiocarcinoma. Endosc Ultrasound 2013; 2(2):71–6.

62. Cârțână ET, Gheonea DI, Săftoiu A. Advances in endoscopic ultrasound imaging of colorectal diseases. World J Gastroenterol 2016;22(5):1756–66.

63. Harewood GC, Wiersema MJ, Nelson H, et al. A prospective, blinded assessment of the impact of preoperative staging on the management of rectal cancer. Gastroenterology 2002;123:24–32.

64. Randomised trial of surgery alone versus radiotherapy followed by surgery for potentially operable locally advanced rectal cancer. Medical Research Council Rectal Cancer Working Party. Lancet 1996;348:1605–10.

65. Worrell S, Horvath K, Blakemore T, et al. Endorectal ultrasound detection of focal carcinoma within rectal adenomas. Am J Surg 2004;187:625–9 [discussion: 629].

66. Marone P, de Bellis M, D'Angelo V, et al. Role of endoscopic ultrasonography in the loco-regional staging of patients with rectal cancer. World J Gastrointest Endosc 2015;7(7):688–701.

67. Puli SR, Reddy JB, Bechtold ML, et al. Accuracy of endoscopic ultrasound to diagnose nodal invasion by rectal cancers: a meta-analysis and systematic review. Ann Surg Oncol 2009;16:1255–65.

68. Cârțână ET, Pârvu D, Săftoiu A. Endoscopic ultrasound: current role and future perspectives in managing rectal cancer patients. J Gastrointestin Liver Dis 2011;20:407–13.

69. Knight CS, Eloubeidi MA, Crowe R, et al. Utility of endoscopic ultrasound-guided fine-needle aspiration in the diagnosis and staging of colorectal carcinoma. Diagn Cytopathol 2013;41(12):1031–7.

70. Shami VM, Parmar KS, Waxman I. Clinical impact of endoscopic ultrasound and endoscopic ultrasound-guided fine-needle aspiration in the management of rectal carcinoma. Dis Colon Rectum 2004;47:59–65.

71. Valero M, Robles-Medranda C. Endoscopic ultrasound in oncology: An update of clinical applications in the gastrointestinal tract. World journal of gastrointestinal endoscopy 2017;9(6):243.

72. Gall TM, Markar SR, Jackson D, et al. Mini-probe ultrasonography for the staging of colon cancer: a systematic review and meta-analysis. Colorectal Dis 2014;16. O1–O8.

73. Malmstrøm ML, Săftoiu A, Vilmann P, et al. Endoscopic ultrasound for staging of colonic cancer proximal to the rectum: a systematic review and meta-analysis. Endosc Ultrasound 2016;5(5):307–14.

74. Castro-Pocas FM, Dinis-Ribeiro M, Rocha A, et al. Colon carcinoma staging by endoscopic ultrasonography miniprobes. Endosc Ultrasound 2017;6(4):245–51.

75. Giovannini M, Seitz JF, Sfedj D, et al. Transanorectal ultrasonography in the evaluation of extension and the monitoring of epidermoid cancers of the anus treated by radiation or chemotherapy. Gastroenterol Clin Biol 1992;16:994–8.

76. Giovannini M, Bardou VJ, Barclay R, et al. Anal carcinoma: prognostic value of endorectal ultrasound (ERUS). Results of a prospective multicenter study. Endoscopy 2001;33(3):231–6.

77. Tarantino D, Bernstein MA. Endoanal ultrasound in the staging and management of squamous-cell carcinoma of the anal canal: potential implications of a new ultrasound staging system. Dis Colon Rectum 2002;45(1):16–22.

78. Săftoiu A. State-of-the-art imaging techniques in endoscopic ultrasound. World J Gastroenterol 2011;17:691–6.

79. Waage JE, Havre RF, Odegaard S, et al. Endorectal elastography in the evaluation of rectal tumours. Colorectal Dis 2011;13:1130–7.

80. Miyata T, Kitano M, Sakamoto H, et al. Role of contrast-enhanced harmonic EUS in differentiating malignant from benign lymphadenopathy. Gastrointest Endosc 2013;77.

Endoscopic Resection of Early Luminal Cancer

Hyuk Soon Choi, MD, PhD[a], Joo Ha Hwang, MD, PhD[b],*

KEYWORDS

- Endoscopic resection • Endoscopic submucosal dissection
- Endoscopic mucosal resection • Early luminal cancer

KEY POINTS

- Early-stage luminal cancers confined to the mucosal layer or superficial submucosal layer can be cured by endoscopic resection.
- Techniques for endoscopic resection include endoscopic mucosal resection (EMR), endoscopic submucosal dissection (ESD), and endoscopic full-thickness resection (EFTR).
- Various devices are available for performing endoscopic resection. It is essential to be familiary with and use the correct device(s).
- It is essential to understand the potential complications from endoscopic resection and know how to manage any complication that may arise.

INTRODUCTION

For most cancers, early detection is the most important factor in curing the disease. In the case of gastrointestinal (GI) cancers, early diagnosis through endoscopy and early detection through screening increase the cure rate. The survival rate for early-stage gastric and colorectal cancer is reported to be more than 90%.[1,2] In the past, detecting early-stage cancers through endoscopy still necessitated open or laparoscopic surgery for removal. However, advances in therapeutic endoscopy now enable the resection of early-stage GI cancers using endoscopic techniques, when appropriate.

Endoscopic resection (ER) is a minimally invasive technique for removing early cancer or precancerous lesions from the GI tract. GI endoscopic surgery can improve the quality of life of patients and reduce healthcare costs by allowing them to forgo open or laparoscopic surgery for early-stage cancers. The detection of early-stage GI cancer and the advancement of ER techniques have led to a significant increase in cure rates. This has allowed for the successful treatment of many patients with early-stage

[a] Korea University College of Medicine, Stanford University Medicine, Korea University Anam Hospital, Goryeodae-ro 73, Seongbuk-gu, Seoul 02841, South Korea; [b] Division of Gastroenterology and Hepatology, Department of Medicine, Stanford University Medicine, Stanford Hospital, 300 Pasteur Drive, H0268, MC: 5244, Stanford, CA 94305, USA
* Corresponding author,
E-mail address: jooha@stanford.edu

Gastrointest Endoscopy Clin N Am 34 (2024) 51–78
https://doi.org/10.1016/j.giec.2023.07.002
1052-5157/24/© 2023 Elsevier Inc. All rights reserved.

cancer, leading to a better prognosis and a reduced risk of recurrence. Initially, before the development of the endoscopic electrosurgical knifes, cancers were removed using only endoscopic mucosal resection (EMR), a method that uses a snare. However, the size of the tumor that could be resected was limited by the size of the snare, so it was generally used for tumors 2 cm or smaller because *en bloc* resection is a requirement for an oncologic resection. To address the challenges of EMR, the development of advanced endoscopic surgery instruments such as electrosurgical knives and electrosurgical units (ESUs) has made it possible to perform endoscopic submucosal dissection (ESD). Compared with EMR, ESD allows for the removal of larger and deeper tumors with greater precision, expanding the range of cases that can be treated. Initially used for stomach cancer, ESD has since been applied to other regions of the GI tract, such as the esophagus, duodenum, and colon, offering improved treatment options for patients with dysplasia and early-stage GI cancers.

Depending on the location within the GI tract, different indications and methods are used for ESD. Recently, submucosal tunneling ER (STER) using the tunnel method and endoscopic full-thickness resection (EFTR), a form of hybrid ER, has also been used to resect subepithelial GI tumors. In this article, the principles and procedural methods of EMR/ESD/STER/EFTR for ER for each GI organ with are explained. No matter what method is used, the most important aspect of an oncologic resection is to obtain an *en bloc* R0 resection. The outcomes of ER and the response to postprocedural complications will also be addressed.

NATURE OF THE PROBLEM

ER techniques, such as EMR and ESD, have become popular due to the minimally invasive nature compared with traditional surgical methods. These procedures have revolutionized the treatment of early-stage GI cancers and other benign or premalignant lesions. Despite its numerous advantages, there are inherent challenges associated with the procedure.

The nature of the GI tract presents several technical difficulties during ER. First, the complex and variable anatomy of the GI tract may pose challenges during the procedure, especially in areas with tight angulations or difficult-to-reach locations such as the duodenum and ascending colon. Second, large, flat, or irregularly shaped lesions may be challenging to resect completely. Moreover, lesions in certain locations, such as cardia, pylorus, or ileocecal valve, may be more difficult to manage endoscopically. Third, ER, particularly ESD, requires a high level of expertise and has a long learning curve. Inadequate training or limited experience can lead to incomplete resections or increased risk of complications.

Although ER is minimally invasive, it can still lead to complications such as perforation, which is more likely in ESD than EMR, intraoperative and delayed bleeding, rare instances of postoperative infection, and stricture formation after extensive resections for esophagus or colon cancer. Moreover, ER has limitations like the potential for incomplete removal of larger or complex lesions, being mainly suited for early-stage GI cancers rather than advanced ones, and a limited capacity to evaluate and address lymph node metastasis. To overcome these complications and limitations, it is important to understand the characteristics and anatomy of each region of the GI tract and to be familiar with the relevant indications and techniques to avoid complications.

ANATOMY OF THE GASTROINTESTINAL WALL FOR ENDOSCOPIC RESECTION

A comprehensive understanding of the structural characteristics of each GI organ, particularly those related to the GI tract wall, is essential for performing successful

ERs. Even within the GI tract, there are differences in the wall structure of the esophagus, stomach, duodenum, and large intestine. Here, we aim to explain the anatomic characteristics of each organ relevant to ER techniques, such as ESD. **Fig. 1** shows the cross-sectional anatomy of various locations within the GI tract.

1. Esophagus

   The esophagus consists of four layers: the mucosa (innermost), the submucosa, the muscularis propria, and the adventitia (outermost). The mucosa is composed of epithelial cells (M1), a thin layer of connective tissue called the lamina propria (M2) and a thin layer of muscle called the muscularis mucosae (M3). In the case of squamous cell invasion, there is a possibility of nodal metastasis from M3 invasion onward. The submucosa is the layer beneath the mucosa, made up of connective tissue, blood vessels, nerves, and glands that produce mucus to lubricate the esophagus during swallowing.[3,4]

2. Stomach

   The mucosa of stomach is the most superficial layer of the gastric wall and comprises three sublayers: epithelium, lamina propria, and muscularis mucosae.

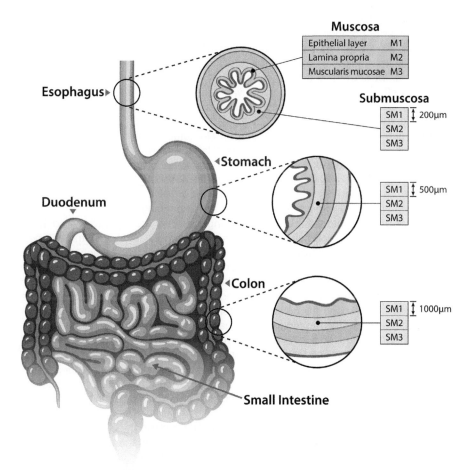

Fig. 1. Anatomy of the gastrointestinal tract for endoscopic resection.

The submucosa is a layer of dense irregular connective tissue situated beneath the mucosa. It contains blood vessels, lymphatic vessels, and nerves. Unlike esophageal ESD, successful gastric ESD requires a greater understanding of the submucosa in the gastric wall structure because the likelihood of lymph node metastasis is related to the depth of submucosal invasion of adenocarcinoma in gastric cancer. The submucosa layer is divided into three parts based on the depth of invasion in increments of 500 μm: Sm1 (less than 500 μm), Sm2 (greater than 500 μm but <1000 μm), and Sm3 (greater than 1000 μm). Proper assessment of these layers and adherence to ESD criteria can lead to successful treatment of early-stage GI neoplasms, reduced complications, and improved patient outcomes. In general, the submucosal layer of the gastric antrum has fewer blood vessels, and the connective tissue is less dense, making dissection relatively easy. On the other hand, the submucosal layer of the gastric body and fundus contains more fibrous tissue and a higher concentration of blood vessels than the antrum, making the dissection of the submucosal layer more challenging.

3. Duodenum

Owing to the duodenum's thin wall, anatomic curvature, and proximity to major blood vessels and the pancreaticobiliary system, the risk of complications, such as perforation and bleeding, is significantly higher compared with ER performed in the stomach or esophagus. Performing ER (such as ESD) in the duodenum requires a detailed understanding of its complex anatomy, including the ampulla of Vater and other important structures that can affect the safety and efficacy of the procedure as well as special caution due to the duodenum's proximity to vital organs such as the pancreas and bile duct.

4. Colon/rectum (colorectum)

ESD can be used to treat early-stage colorectal cancers or large polyps by excising the lesion from the submucosal layer, keeping the muscularis propria intact. In the context of colon ESD, understanding the submucosal layer is crucial, as this is the primary target for dissection. The colon is attached to the posterior abdominal wall through the mesentery, a fold of the peritoneum that supports and anchors the colon. The ascending and descending colon have a retroperitoneal position, meaning that they are fixed to the posterior abdominal wall, whereas the transverse and sigmoid colon are intraperitoneal and have more mobility due to their longer mesenteric attachments. The cecum is the widest part of the colon and has a thinner wall compared with other regions of the colon. ESD in the cecum requires careful dissection to avoid perforation. In addition, the ileocecal valve, the junction between the small intestine and the colon, is anatomically complex, with folds and curves that may make the procedure more challenging. Limited space and maneuverability in the ileocecal valve area may make it more difficult to obtain an optimal endoscopic view and maintain a stable position during the procedure. Appropriate scope handling and patient positioning can help overcome these challenges. The transverse colon and sigmoid colon have longer mesenteries, which provide greater mobility and require caution during endoscopic procedures.

It is important to avoid putting undue tension on the mesentery and its blood supply to prevent complications such as ischemia or damage to the surrounding structures. Owing to the lower blood flow in part of colon compared with other abdominal organs, colonoscopy poses a risk for colon ischemia, which can have multiple causes such as splanchnic circulation impairment, bowel preparation, sedative drugs, bowel wall ischemia due to insufflation or baro-trauma, and the introduction of the endoscope.[5]

The rectum is located in the pelvic cavity and is surrounded by various pelvic structures, such as the prostate or uterus, seminal vesicles, and urinary bladder. During ESD in the rectum, it is essential to consider these neighboring structures to avoid damaging them inadvertently. In addition, the rectum has a relatively consistent diameter and straight configuration, making endoscope navigation and lesion visualization easier. However, its more abundant blood supply may pose a higher risk of bleeding, requiring extra care to avoid injury to larger vessels. The rectal wall is generally thicker than the colonic wall. This thickness difference affects the dissection process during ESD. In the rectum, the thicker wall may provide more stability and reduce the risk of perforation, whereas in the colon, the thinner wall requires a more delicate approach to prevent accidental damage to muscle layer.

INDICATIONS FOR ENDOSCOPIC RESECTION

Indication for Endoscopic Resection of Esophageal Cancer

Early-stage esophageal cancer confined to the mucosal layer or submucosal layer is referred to as superficial esophageal cancer. Most of these cases are in the initial stages, allowing for long-term survival after treatment. The detection rate of early esophageal cancer is increasing in some regions, and advancements in endoscopic local treatments are significantly improving esophageal cancer care.[6]

One of the most important considerations in endoscopic treatment of esophageal cancer is that the histopathological characteristics are significantly different from those of gastric cancer. Although dividing the mucosal layer into M1, M2, and M3 in gastric cancer may not be very meaningful, it is extremely important in squamous cell esophageal cancer.[7] The reason for the detailed classification of the mucosal layer in esophageal cancer is that the risk of lymph node metastasis dramatically increases with involvement of M3.

In esophageal cancer, SM1 refers to up to 200 μm (**Fig. 1**). The American Gastroenterological Association (AGA) Institute Clinical Practice Update provides separate ESD indications for squamous cell carcinoma and Barrett's esophagus[8] (**Table 1**).

Table 1
Indication for esophageal endoscopic submucosal dissection in the United States

Condition	Indications for Esophageal ESD
Squamous cell carcinoma	High-grade dysplasia (HGD) to well-differentiated (G1) or moderately differentiated (G2) squamous cell carcinoma
	Paris 0–II lesions
	Absolute indications: m1–m2 involvement with two-thirds or less of the esophageal circumference
	Expanded indications: m3 or SM < 200 μm involvement, any size, clinically N0
Barrett's esophagus	HGD to moderately differentiated (G1 or G2) T1a (m1–m3) lesions ≥ 15 mm (not amenable to *en bloc* resection by EMR)
	Large or bulky area of nodularity
	Equivocal preprocedure histology
	Intramucosal carcinoma
	Suspected superficial submucosal invasion
	Recurrent dysplasia
	EMR specimen showing invasive carcinoma with positive margins

Recently, the Japan Gastroenterological Endoscopy Society (JGES) provided guidelines for esophageal cancer ESD, which are based on the depth of invasion, size, and circumferential extent. For clinical T1a-epithelium/lamina propria mucosa (N0M0) cancer, ER can be performed for non-circumferential lesions, whereas for whole circumferential lesions, ER is recommended for those up to 5 cm and surgical resection or chemoradiotherapy for those larger than 5 cm. If an esophageal cancer is staged as T1a-MM or T1b-SM1, ER can be performed for non-circumferential lesions, followed by pathologic assessment to determine if the resection was curative. For circumferential lesions, surgical resection or chemoradiotherapy is recommended.[9]

Indication for Endoscopic Resection of Gastric Cancer

The indications for gastric ESD are generally based on the risk of lymph node metastasis and the likelihood of achieving complete resection. In gastric cancer ESD, absolute indications and expanded criteria have been suggested in Japan by Gotoda, and various countries have presented ESD indications suitable by their respective national gastroenterological endoscopy societies[8,10] (**Tables 2** and **3**).

The criteria for lesions that can be determined by preoperative endoscopy are somewhat subjective. It is difficult to accurately distinguish between M cancer (mucosal cancer) and SM (submucosal) cancer through endoscopic findings alone. Although endoscopic ultrasound (EUS) can be used to assess the depth of invasion before EMR or ESD, it is not always capable of accurately diagnosing very small submucosal invasions. As a result, conducting EUS before EMR/ESD can provide useful information, but it is not considered an essential prerequisite for these procedures. In gastric cancer, ESD is indicated for absolute indications including intramucosal

Table 2
Indication for gastric cancer endoscopic submucosal dissection

Depth	Mucosal cancer				Submucosal cancer	
	Ulceration		No ulceration		Sm1(invasion depth ≤ 500um)	Sm2,3 (Invasion depth ≥ 500 um)
Lesion size	≤2cm	>2cm	≤3cm	>3cm	≤3cm	Any size
Differentiated carcinoma						
Undifferentiated carcinoma						

□ Guideline criteria for EMR　　■ Surgery

■ Expanded criteria for ESD　　□ possible surgery or ESD

Table 3
American Gastroenterological Association recommendation for gastric cancer endoscopic submucosal dissection

Indications	Type	Differentiation	Size	Ulceration	Invasion
Absolute	Mucosal adenocarcinoma (and lesions with HGD), intestinal type	G1 or G2	≤ 2 cm	No	mucosa
Expanded	Adenocarcinoma, intestinal type	G1 or G2	Any size	No	mucosa
	Adenocarcinoma, intestinal type	G1 or G2	-	-	SM < 500 μm
	Adenocarcinoma, intestinal type	G1 or G2	≥ 3 cm	Yes	mucosa
	Adenocarcinoma, diffuse type	G3 or G4	≤ 2 cm	No	mucosa

gastric adenocarcinoma (cT1a) with differentiated histology, lesion size ≤ 2 cm, no evidence of ulceration (UL0), and no lymphovascular invasion, whereas expanded indications encompass larger lesions, undifferentiated histology, and submucosal invasion up to 500 μm with favorable prognostic factors.

It is essential to note that the indications for gastric ESD may vary among countries and institutions, as they are influenced by factors such as clinical expertise and local guidelines. In addition, patient factors, such as age, overall health, and comorbidities, should be considered when determining the suitability of gastric ESD.

Indication for Endoscopic Resection of Duodenal Lesions

EMR or ESD can be performed in the duodenum, but it is less common and more technically challenging compared with gastric or esophageal ESD. The indications for duodenal ESD include early-stage duodenal cancers or precancerous lesions, such as large adenomas, which are limited to the mucosa or superficial submucosa layers without evidence of lymph node metastasis or distant metastasis.

However, due to the duodenum's thin wall, anatomic curvature and proximity to major blood vessels and the pancreaticobiliary system, the risk of complications, such as perforation and bleeding, is significantly higher compared with ESD performed in the stomach or esophagus. Therefore, the decision to perform ESD in the duodenum should be made on a case-by-case basis, considering factors such as lesion size, location, histology, and the patient's overall health. In addition, the procedure should be performed by experienced endoscopists who are skilled in managing potential complications.

Indications for Endoscopic Resection of Colorectal Cancers

EMR is typically suitable for lesions smaller than 20 mm and those with a low risk of lymph node metastasis. ESD is a more advanced technique used to achieve *en bloc* resection of larger lesions or those difficult to remove with EMR, such as lesions with significant submucosal fibrosis. ESD involves the dissection of the submucosal layer beneath the lesion, allowing for more precise removal of the tumor while minimizing the risk of recurrence. ESD is indicated for lesions with superficial submucosal invasion, minimal lymph node metastasis risk, and lateral spreading tumors (LSTs) larger than 20 mm. The AGA has published indications for colon ESD, which are summarized in **Table 4**.[8]

The choice between EMR and ESD depends on factors such as lesion size, location, morphology, and the endoscopist's skill level. If the lesion to be resected is suspected

Table 4
American Gastroenterological Association recommendation for colorectal endoscopic submucosal dissection

Risk Factor	Description (Paris)	Size
En bloc Resection for Lesions at Risk for Submucosally Invasive Cancer:		
Type V Kudo pit pattern	-	-
Depressed component	0–IIc	-
Complex morphology	0–Is or 0–IIa + Is	-
Rectosigmoid location	-	-
Nongranular LST (adenomas)	-	≥ 20 mm
Granular LST (adenomas)	-	≥ 30 mm
Residual or recurrent adenomas		

to be a malignancy, it is essential that the lesion be resected *en bloc* for histopathologic evaluation. The decision to perform either ESD or EMR should take this into consideration. Both techniques aim to provide effective treatment while preserving the patient's quality of life and minimizing complications.

The indications for ER of malignant colorectal polyps may vary depending on whether the polyp is pedunculated or non-pedunculated. Pedunculated polyps are polyps with a stalk, whereas non-pedunculated polyps do not have a stalk and are sessile or flat.

According to the US Multi-Society Task Force on Colorectal Cancer (the American Society for Gastrointestinal Endoscopy (ASGE), the American College of Gastroenterology (ACG), and the AGA) guidelines on the management of malignant colorectal polyps, non-pedunculated malignant polyps should be considered high risk for residual or recurrent cancer if they have any of the following features: poor tumor differentiation, lymphovascular invasion, submucosal invasion depth greater than 1 mm, tumor involvement of the cautery margin, or tumor budding. For pedunculated malignant polyps, the ASGE guidelines recommend that they are considered high risk for residual or recurrent cancer if they have poor tumor differentiation, lymphovascular invasion, or tumor within 1 mm of the resection margin.[11]

In general, ER (either EMR or ESD) can be considered for malignant colorectal polyps that meet certain criteria, such as tumor is resected *en bloc*, no evidence of deep submucosal invasion, no evidence of lymphovascular invasion, and negative resection margins. However, for polyps with high-risk features or larger size, surgical resection with lymph node dissection may be recommended.

PROCEDURAL APPROACH
Endoscopic Mucosal Resection

EMR is primarily used for the removal of polypoid tumors in the GI tract. However, recent advances have led to the utilization of modified EMR techniques such as piecemeal EMR, EMR-L, and EMR with cap-assisted technique (EMR-C) for lesions with LSTs and fibrosis.

EMR is one of the most commonly used resection techniques for the safe and effective removal of tumors smaller than 20 mm. However, for lesions larger than 20 mm, such as non-pedunculated flat adenomatous polyps, LSTs, submucosal tumors, lesions in difficult-to-access locations due to flexures or folds, lesions with accompanying fibrosis due to prior biopsies or partial resections, and locally recurrent cases following ER, conventional EMR may have a relatively low *en bloc* resection rate. In such cases, hybrid ESD or ESD should be considered. Generally, for polyps larger than 20 mm, endoscopic piecemeal resection or ESD should be considered based on the possibility of malignancy.

1. Conventional endoscopic mucosal resection

Conventional-EMR is a method of resection using an endoscope after injecting submucosal injection solution and using a snare. The submucosal injection of the polyp creates a cushion space between the mucosa and the muscularis propria, which can prevent perforation, and there is also a mechanical compression effect on the microvessels of the submucosal layer, allowing for safer removal of the polyp. In addition, if resection is difficult due to the colonic flexure of the GI tract, or if the lesion is not clearly distinguishable from the normal mucosa, making it difficult to capture with adequate margins, submucosal injection can help facilitate polyp resection more easily. Various submucosal injection materials are used, such as normal saline, glycerin, hyaluronic acid, sodium alginate, and hydroxyethyl starch. Generally, solutions containing epinephrine and a small amount of indigo carmine or methylene blue are used to reduce the risk of bleeding and to visualize the injection site. The submucosal solution is preferably injected into the proximal part of the polyp so that the lesion swells in front of the endoscope tip, making it easier to capture, and efforts should be made to inject at an angle of 30 to 45° to penetrate the mucosal barrier as close to vertical as possible. When injecting the submucosal solution into the proximal part of the polyp, slowly pull the needle back while pointing it downward, so the lesion moves to the center of the swelling, making resection easier **(Fig. 2)**.

2. Modified EMR (EMR-Cap/EMR-Ligation)

If the polyp is not captured at once due to factors such as lesion location or swelling shape after submucosal solution injection, EMR using modified method can be considered. Cap-assisted EMR (EMR-C), which involves applying a cap with a snare to the endoscope tip and sufficiently aspirating the lesion into the cap, and ligation-assisted EMR (EMR-Ligation, EMR-L), which uses a cap with a rubber band to capture the lesion and resect it with a snare, can be tried. However, using these devices has the disadvantage of making it difficult to control the capture depth, so they are typically used in rectal lesions with thicker submucosal layers. For lesions with fibrosis where mucosal swelling does not occur well, there is underwater EMR, which is performed by filling the colonic lumen with water instead of air and without using

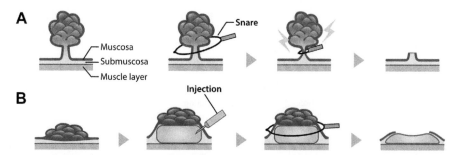

Fig. 2. Conventional endoscopic mucosal resection. (*A*) Cold snare resection without submucosal injection. (*B*) EMR after submucosal injection.

submucosal injection solution. EMR is a minimally invasive technique used to remove GI neoplasms. Several EMR techniques have been developed to treat various types of lesions, EMR-C, and EMR-L.

1. EMR with cap-assisted technique:

    EMR-C, also known as cap-assisted EMR, involves the use of a transparent cap attached to the tip of the endoscope. The cap assists in stabilizing the lesion and provides better visualization. A snare is premounted to the distal end of the cap and advanced to the lesion. After marking the lesion and injecting a solution into the submucosal layer, the lesion is then suctioned into the cap and the snare is then closed around the base of the lesion. The lesion is resected using electrosurgical current, and the specimen is retrieved. This technique allows for easier manipulation of the lesion and can improve the resection rate (**Fig. 3**).

2. EMR with ligation:

    EMR-L, also known as band ligation-assisted EMR, is a technique that combines endoscopic variceal ligation with EMR. After marking the lesion and injecting a solution into the submucosal layer, a ligation device is used to place a rubber band around the base of the lesion, capturing and strangulating it. The lesion, along with a portion of the surrounding tissue, is then resected using a snare and electrosurgical current. The specimen is retrieved by cutting the rubber band (**Fig. 4**). EMR-L is particularly useful for the resection of larger and sessile lesions, as the ligation process reduces the risk of bleeding and perforation.

Each of these EMR techniques has its advantages and limitations, and the choice of the technique depends on factors such as lesion size, location, and morphology as well as the endoscopist's experience and preference. In general, all methods of EMR are limited to lesions less than 20 mm in diameter to achieve an *en bloc* resection.

Hybrid Endoscopic Submucosal Dissection

Hybrid ESD is a technique in which the lesion is first marked, submucosal injection is performed and then a full circumferential incision is made around the lesion with an electrosurgical knife to create a margin around the lesion. Limited submucosal dissection is performed to expose the submucosal layer circumferentially as well as any areas under the lesion where there is submucosal fibrosis limiting the lifting of the mucosal surface. This step is then followed by injecting a solution into the submucosal layer to elevate the remainder of the mucosal lesion, creating a cushion between the mucosal and deeper layers. After the injection, the lesion is resected using a snare, and the specimen is retrieved. The circumferential incision step allows for precise control of the resection margins and sets the depth of the resection, which may reduce the risk of incomplete resection and local recurrence (**Fig. 5**).

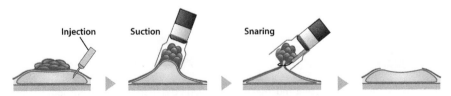

Fig. 3. Endoscopic mucosal resection with cap-assisted technique (EMR-C).

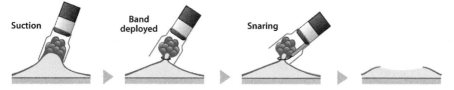

Fig. 4. Endoscopic mucosal resection with ligation (EMR-L).

Endoscopic Submucosal Dissection

ESD was introduced in Japan in the 1990s for the curative resection of early gastric cancer (EGC). Compared with EMR, ESD allows for relatively unrestricted *en bloc* resection regardless of size, location, and shape. It is currently actively used for the complete resection of benign and malignant tumors in the GI tract, including the esophagus, stomach, duodenum, and colon. Regardless of the specific ESD technique used, the fundamental principles of the procedure remain consistent. These basic steps include marking the lesion, administering a submucosal injection, creating a mucosal incision around the lesion, and dissecting the underlying submucosal tissue. By adhering to these core principles, physicians can adapt their approach based on the unique needs of the patient while maintaining the effectiveness of the treatment (**Fig. 6**).

Once the examination and setting plan for the procedure have been completed, it is helpful to perform mental image preparation for the ESD procedure before starting. After predicting the lesion's location, size, distribution of blood vessels in the submucosal layer, and fibrosis, consider which knife to use, which angle to start the mucosal incision to facilitate visibility in case of bleeding, and where to begin submucosal dissection to maximize the exposure of the submucosal layer with the help of gravity. It is recommended to create a somewhat specific scenario and simulate it.

1. Lesion confirmation

    Before ER of GI lesions, it is essential to accurately confirm the patient's lesion status. Chromoendoscopy using indigo carmine to paint the lesion has been used to accurately assess the margins of the lesion, but recently, image-enhancing endoscopy/electronic chromoendoscopy such as narrow band image (NBI), i-SCAN, and flexible spectral imaging color enhancement have been demonstrated to accurately determine the lesion margins and characterize the lesion. Confirming the lesion helps to accurately determine whether ER is indicated by evaluating the presence of ulcers and lesion size.

2. Choices of ESD devices

    a. Electrosurgical knife

        First, it is necessary to decide which knife to use for the ESD resection. There are various ESD knives currently available, each with its own advantages and disadvantages, and new products are constantly being developed and released.[12,13] Currently, there is no one knife that has the ability to

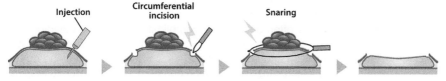

Fig. 5. Hybrid ESD.

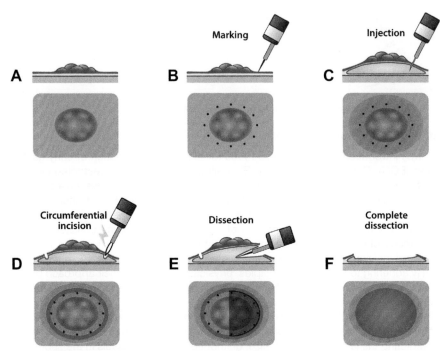

Fig. 6. Endoscopic submucosal dissection. (*A*) Lesion confirmation. (*B*) Marking. (*C*) Submucosal injection. (*D*) Circumferential incision. (*E*) Dissection. (*F*) Complete dissection after retrieval of tissue is resected.

do it all. Therefore, it is important to choose the most appropriate knife for each step of the procedure, and most importantly, whether the operator can handle it comfortably and safely. Because the usage methods differ for each knife, the operator should be well versed in the characteristics and advantages/disadvantages of the knife before starting the procedure. There is little research on which knife is suitable for beginners and has fewer complications. Morphologically, knives can be divided into insulated and non-insulated knives, but recently, knives that combine the advantages of both have also been released (**Fig. 7**).

b. Electrosurgical unit

A thorough understanding of the ESU is crucial when performing ESD. Operators intending to perform ESD should be well versed in the principles of electrosurgery, particularly the characteristics and application of various cutting and coagulation settings. This theoretic preparation is essential for addressing various situations encountered during ESD and EMR, such as difficulty in dissection due to tissue carbonization, fibrosis with scars, and ineffective resection due to increased resistance in the submucosal layer with abundant adipose tissue, by changing the cutting and coagulation settings.

c. Endoscopic caps/hoods

The ESD procedure often encounters complications such as bleeding and perforation. To reduce these complications, it is important to closely observe the incision and dissection surfaces. However, depending on the location of the lesion, close observation can be challenging due to respiration and cardiac movement. In such cases, attaching a transparent cap to

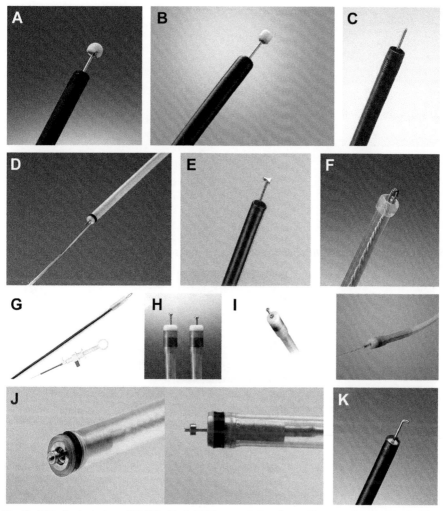

Fig. 7. ESD electroknives. (*A*) IT knife 2 (With permission from Olympus Corporation). (*B*) IT knife nano (With permission from Olympus Corporation). (*C*) Needle knife (With permission from Olympus Corporation). (*D*) Splash knife (Splash M-KnifeTM (PENTAX Medical, HOYA Corporation, Tokyo, Japan). With permission from PENTAX Medical, HOYA Corporation). (*E*) Triangle tip knife (With permission from Olympus Corporation). (*F*). Flex knife (With permission from Olympus Corporation). (*G*) Universal knife (ESD-knife. With permission from MTW Endoskopie Manufaktur). (*H*) Dual knife (With permission from Olympus Corporation). (*I*) Dual knife J (Water jet, With permission from Olympus Corporation). (*J*) Splash M-KnifeTM (PENTAX Medical, HOYA Corporation, Tokyo, Japan). With permission from PENTAX Medical, HOYA Corporation. (*K*) Hook knife (rotatable, With permission from Olympus Corporation).

the end of the endoscope allows a close approach to the lesion, maintaining a consistent distance of about 3 to 4 mm between the lesion's incision and dissection surfaces, greatly aiding in the close observation (**Fig. 8**).
  d. Hemostatic devices
      Bleeding can occur at any stage of the ESD procedure. For instance, it can occur during the process of marking around the lesion using electric

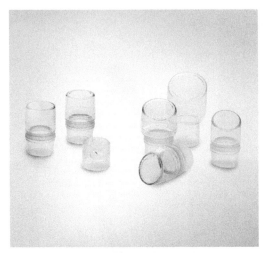

Fig. 8. Endoscopic caps (With permission from Olympus Corporation).

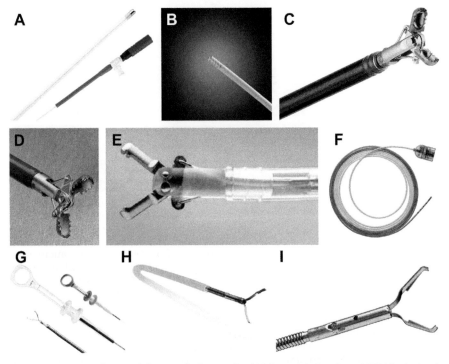

Fig. 9. Hemostatic devices. (*A*) Coagulation probe (With permission from MTW Endoskopie Manufaktur). (*B*) Injection Gold Probe TM (Image provided courtesy of Boston Scientific. ©2023 Boston Scientific Corporation or its affiliates. All rights reserved). (*C*) Coagrasper (With permission from Olympus Corporation). (*D*) Hot biopsy forceps (Image provided courtesy of Boston Scientific. ©2023 Boston Scientific Corporation or its affiliates. All rights reserved). (*E*) Hemostat-Y (HemoStat-YTM (PENTAX Medical, HOYA Corporation, Tokyo, Japan). With permission from PENTAX Medical, HOYA Corporation). (*F*) Argon plasma coagulation probe (ERBE, Germany). (*G*) EZ Clip (With permission from Olympus Corporation). (*H*) QuickPro (With permission from Olympus Corporation). (*I*) Resolution clip (Image provided courtesy of Boston Scientific. ©2023 Boston Scientific Corporation or its affiliates. All rights reserved).

coagulation current or argon plasma coagulation (APC), the submucosal injection process, the process of making an incision around the lesion, and the process of performing submucosal dissection. When bleeding occurs, it is important to know which hemostatic device to use (**Fig. 9**).

3. Marking

Various methods, such as a cutting knife or APC, can be used to mark the cutting line for lesion resection. Typically, marks are made on the normal mucosa about 5 mm to 1 cm away from the lesion's border using a coagulation current.

4. Submucosal injection

The submucosal injection is performed 2 to 3 mm outside the marked resection area. Typically, the injection is started from the distal part of the lesion or the difficult to resect part in the endoscopic view, then the incision is made, and the injection fluid is inserted toward the proximal side, followed by the incision. However, this can vary depending on the location of the lesion. The angle of the injection needle should be approximately 45 to 70° in the stomach and 30 to 45° in the colon. If the submucosal layer does not swell up well, it is usually because the injection needle is inserted too deeply. In this case, it is effective to pull the needle slightly toward the mucosal layer and inject the solution. Injections are usually made in multiple locations, with 1 to 5 cc injection in each location.

5. Circumferential incision and dissection

Understanding the anatomic structure of the GI tract is important for maintaining appropriate incision depth during mucosal incision and submucosal dissection. Most patients maintain a left lateral decubitus position during endoscopic procedures, so it is crucial to understand the direction of gravity and perform the incision and dissection in a direction that exposes the submucosal layer easily.

During submucosal dissection, a series of short, straight lines should be used to follow the overall curvature of the GI wall. The dissection plane of the submucosal layer should be kept as close as possible to the endoscopic view using CO_2 control, pushing and pulling, and torque rotation. The depth of dissection should be at the lower one-third of the submucosal layer or at the boundary between the submucosal layer and the muscularis propria, which helps reduce bleeding in ESD. This boundary can only be confirmed during close-up, direct-view dissection. Attaching a transparent cap to the endoscope tip helps with visibility during close dissection and helps induce countertraction when the tip enters the submucosal layer, aiding in dissection. If a vessel likely to bleed is encountered during dissection, coagulation is performed in advance using a coagulation forceps.

6. Tissue fixation and pathology

Accurate confirmation of the final pathology results in ER is important, as it determines whether complete resection has been achieved or additional surgery is needed. Generally, the dissected tissue is fixed and sent for pathology examination. To prevent the tissue margins from curling inward, the tissue is stretched and flattened as much as possible, pinned to a flat Styrofoam piece, and placed in formalin. However, individual differences in stretching technique may affect the results. Overcoming this issue has been the subject of research, but unifying the method through communication between physicians and pathologists at each center is crucial.

Pathologic criteria for endoscopically resected tissue may vary by country, but generally follow the World Health Organization (WHO) guidelines. Early GI cancer ER pathology diagnosis includes the presence or absence of tumor invasion in the resection margins, determining complete resection, and histologic type, invasion depth, tumor size, ulcer, lymphatic, and vascular invasion, which are known risk factors for lymph node and distant metastasis. The results, except for histologic type, are usually indicated by agreed on terms, numbers, or presence/absence, making it easy to standardize among hospitals and medical centers. However, there may be confusion regarding histologic type and histologic differentiation. In this regard, ongoing communication between the endoscopist and the pathologist is necessary.

Endoscopic Full-Thickness Resection

EFTR is a method of resecting the entire layer of the GI wall surrounding the tumor. Initially developed and mainly used to remove GI subepithelial tumors (SETs), it has also been applied in cases of GI luminal/mucosal cancers where the indication for ESD is unclear. This technique is particularly useful for early-stage cancers, SETs, and benign tumors that have not yet penetrated the GI wall or metastasized to other parts of the body. EFTR can be a valuable option for patients who are not suitable candidates for surgery due to age or comorbidities. EFTR is a minimally invasive technique used to remove GI luminal tumors, such as those in the stomach, small intestine, and colon (**Fig. 10**).

1. Exposed EFTR
   This method involves cutting the entire gastric wall layer around the tumor and removing it, resulting in an artificial perforation that connects the abdominal cavity to the gastric space. To resolve this issue, the procedure is completed

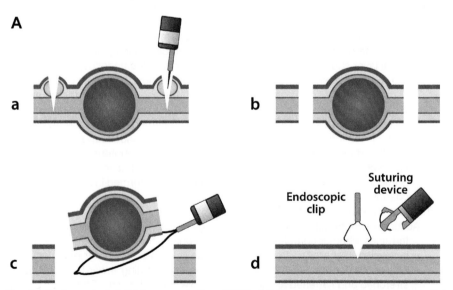

Fig. 10. Endoscopic full-thickness resection (EFTR). (*A*) Exposed EFTR. (*a*) Circumferential incision to the depth of the muscularis propria. (*b*) Intentional perforation to serosal layer. (*c*) Retrieving of resected entire wall including tumor with endoscope. (*d*) Suturing or clipping. (*B*) Nonexposed EFTR (band ligation). (*a*) Lesion confirmation. (*b*) Suction with forceps. (*c*) Band ligation deployed. (*d*) Cutting with snaring. (*C*) Laparoscopic endoscopic cooperative surgery (LECS). (*a*) Circumferential incision to the depth of the muscularis propria. (*b*) Intentional perforation to serosal layer. (*c*) Retrieving of resected entire wall including tumor with laparoscope. (*d*) Suturing with laparoscopic stapler.

B

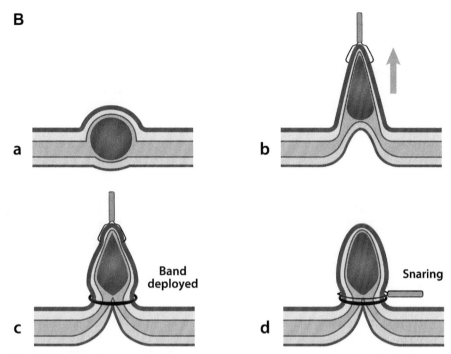

Fig. 10. (*continued*).

by closing the perforation using clips, loops, or endoscopic suturing devices. One consideration during the procedure is that the resected tumor may fall into the abdominal cavity; to prevent this, a grasping forceps can be inserted through a two-channel endoscope to hold the tumor tissue during the resection process. Hybrid methods such as laparoscopic-assisted EFTR (laparoscopic endoscopic cooperative surgery) are also being attempted. In these cases, the possibility of peritoneal infection and tumor cell dissemination due to artificial perforation can be a concern.[14]

2. Nonexposed EFTR (pure EFTR)

This is a surgical method where the tumor is resected without exposing the gastric space to the abdominal cavity. To achieve this, a plication process is included to grasp the folds of the GI wall surrounding the tumor before resection. After the tumor is removed, the resection site must be sutured using an endoscopic suturing device. Theoretically, nonexposed EFTR has many advantages; however, when using a flexible endoscope, there is a limitation to the size of the tumor that can be resected. Moreover, currently, there are no commercially available devices specifically designed for this technique in GI tumors.

The nonexposed EFTR technique involves the creation of a "double-layer" or "pseudo-cavity" to avoid exposing the resected area to the GI lumen. A solution is injected into the submucosal layer to lift the tumor away from the deeper layers, and then a circumferential mucosal incision is made around the tumor. Afterward, the seromuscular layer is incised, completing the full-thickness resection. The defect is closed using endoscopic sutures, clips, or other specialized devices without ever exposing the resected area to the GI lumen.

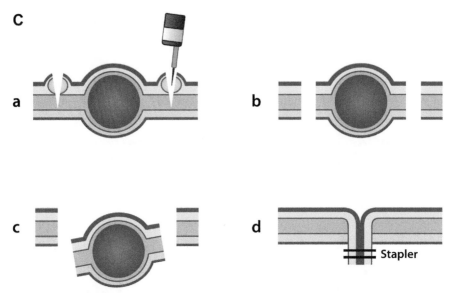

Fig. 10. (*continued*).

EFTR is a promising technique for the management of early-stage GI luminal cancers, providing a minimally invasive alternative to traditional surgery. However, patient selection and endoscopic expertise are crucial factors in determining the success of the procedure.

Submucosal Tunneling Endoscopic Resection/Endoscopic Submucosal Tunneling Dissection

STER was initially developed to resect SETs in the esophagus and gastroesophageal junction.[15] Subsequently, the technique was attempted for tumors in other parts of the GI tract, such as the rectum.[16] Compared with other ER techniques, the advantages of STER include preserving the mucosa, accelerating wound healing, and reducing the risk of infection. Several studies have already demonstrated the safety and efficacy of STER in the treatment of gastric submucosal tumors.[17]

However, there are limitations when using STER in stomach, such as difficulty in accessing lesions in the upper and lower parts of the stomach, and the challenge of removing tumors larger than 4 cm through the mouth. Recently, there have been reports of cases where the STER/endoscopic submucosal tunnel dissection method was used to remove lesions such as EGC and other mucosa cancers when fibrosis was severe or the deep margin was uncertain. In these cases, performing a sufficiently deep dissection during the procedure can enable *en bloc* resection of lesions that may be incompletely resected using the conventional ESD method.[18] The STER procedure for stomach tumors offers several advantages, including minimal invasiveness, preservation of the mucosal layer, and reduced risk of complications (**Fig. 11**).

CHARACTERISTICS OF ENDOSCOPIC RESECTION PROCEDURES BY ORGAN
Esophagus

The esophageal procedure can be carried out following the sequence of the EMR or ESD methods mentioned above. In the case of ESD, the procedure progresses in the order of marking, submucosal injection, circumferential incision, and dissection.

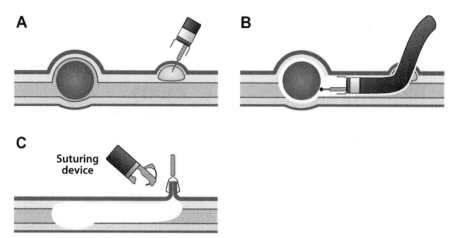

Fig. 11. Submucosal tunneling endoscopic resection (STER). (*A*) Marking and submucosal injection. (*B*) Mucosal incision and tunnel creation. (*C*) Tumor dissection and closure of mucosal incision.

For the esophagus, the esophageal wall is thin, and postoperative stricture may occur, so the procedure should be carried out considering these factors.

The esophagus, a tubular structure, is known to have a high incidence of stricture after ulcer healing in more than 75% of cases with ESD-induced ulcers. One way to prevent stricture is to mark and perform a circumferential incision as close as possible to the lesion. Because squamous cell carcinoma (SCC) esophageal lesions can be clearly observed with Lugol's solution or image-enhancing endoscopy/electronic chromoendoscopy, marking 5 mm outside the lesion and making a circular incision 5 mm outside the marking can bring both sides of the lesion very close, so the range of marking and circumferential incision should be determined with this in mind. If a postoperative stricture is expected, steroid injections can be given during or after the procedure, and/or oral steroids can be prescribed. If a stricture occurs despite these measures, it can be treated with endoscopic balloon dilation, preventive temporary stent insertion, or endoscopic incision (stricturoplasty).

The JGES guidelines reported that the stricture rate when using post-ER stricture prevention strategies was 76% in 45 patients receiving steroid injection therapy, 55% in 44 patients receiving oral steroid therapy, and 71% in 14 patients receiving both steroid injection and oral steroid therapy.[9]

Stomach

For beginners performing ESD for the first time, it is usually recommended to remove small tumors located in the anterior wall of the antrum. Depending on the location of the lesion within the stomach, there are various considerations when performing ESD (**Fig. 12**).

1. Cardia and upper body: The cardia can be a challenging location for beginners, as it may be difficult for the endoscope tip (lens) to get close to the lesion. In addition, the cardia and upper body have a rich vascular supply and thinner gastric walls, making bleeding and perforation more likely, which makes ESD traditionally more difficult. Careful dissection is essential in the cardia and pyloric region, as the gastric wall is concave and may be challenging to operate on. Because it is

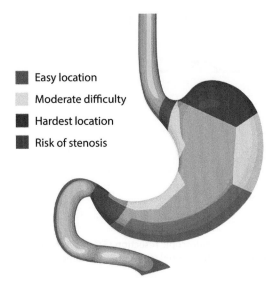

Fig. 12. Difficulty of performing endoscopic submucosal dissection (ESD) by location in the stomach.

difficult to observe the lesion directly, it is important to consider the direction of blood flow during dissection and to keep the lesion as close to the operator as possible in an inverted state. The amount of submucosal injection should be adjusted as needed, as bleeding can occur even with the injection alone. In addition to these location-specific considerations, using both the up-down and left-right levers of the endoscope simultaneously can help access the lesion more effectively.

2. Body: The body presents a higher degree of difficulty for ESD due to the anatomic features, such as abundant blood vessels and fibers, and the difficulty of maneuvering the endoscope. Proper dissection depth and sequence are crucial for successful ESD, and CO_2 insufflation and suctioning should be adjusted during the inverted state to avoid excessive flattening of the lesion and making it difficult to cut and dissect.

The medial longitudinal oblique muscle in the stomach, along with the transverse vasoganglion, forms a fascia-like layer with a network of large blood vessels in the submucosal layer. This structure can cause significant bleeding and difficulty during ESD procedures in the anterior, posterior walls, and the greater curvature of the gastric body. To minimize bleeding and facilitate dissection, it is advised to maintain a dissection depth in the deep submucosal layer, which has fewer fibers and blood vessels. During dissection, thick perforating vessels should be carefully precoagulated using coagulation forceps.

3. Pyloric region: The pyloric region can be particularly challenging due to the proximity of the duodenal bulb. Special attention should be paid to the lesion's location and the submucosal injection to minimize the lesion from bending backward during cutting. Following an ESD procedure in the pylorus area, there is a risk of developing stenosis. Pyloric stenosis can occur due to scarring or fibrosis of the mucosal layer after the resection and healing process. This constriction can lead to difficulty in the passage of food through the pylorus, causing obstructive symptoms such as

vomiting, abdominal pain, and weight loss. To minimize the risk of stenosis, endoscopists should ensure a proper technique during the ESD procedure, focusing on preserving the muscular layer and avoiding excessive tissue removal. In some cases, endoscopic balloon dilation or other interventions may be required to treat stenosis that develops post-ESD.

Colon

Colon ESD poses several challenges depending on the location of the lesion within the colon. Some of the challenges associated with colon ESD based on lesion location include.

1. Cecum: The cecum is a relatively difficult area for ESD due to its thin wall and the presence of the ileocecal valve. Care must be taken to avoid damaging the valve and the risk of perforation is higher in this area.
2. Ascending colon: The ascending colon has a thicker wall compared with other parts of the colon, which can make dissection more challenging. Moreover, the proximity to the hepatic flexure may limit the maneuverability of the endoscope.
3. Transverse colon: The transverse colon can be difficult to access due to its length and mobility. It may be challenging to maintain stable positioning of the endoscope during ESD, and the risk of looping may be higher.
4. Descending colon: The descending colon can be challenging due to its proximity to the splenic flexure, which may limit endoscope maneuverability. In addition, the narrow lumen may make it difficult to maintain adequate visualization during the procedure.
5. Sigmoid colon: The sigmoid colon is highly mobile and has a narrow lumen, which can make ESD more challenging. The risk of looping is higher in this area, and it may be difficult to maintain stable positioning of the endoscope during the procedure.
6. Rectum: The rectum has a thicker wall and a more rigid structure, which can make dissection more challenging. The rectum is easily accessible with a standard colonoscope or upper scope. The risk of perforation during rectal ESD is generally lower than in other parts of the colon due to the thicker wall. However, rectal lesions are more prone to submucosal fibrosis due to prior inflammation or interventions. Fibrosis can make it more difficult to create a proper submucosal cushion and can increase the risk of complications during ESD.

To overcome these challenges, endoscopists must be skilled in maneuvering the endoscope, have a thorough understanding of the colon anatomy, and be able to choose the appropriate ESD technique based on the lesion location. In addition, new overtubes have been developed specifically to assist in stabilization and retraction for colon ESD procedures.

MANAGEMENT FOR ADVERSE EVENTS OF ENDOSCOPIC RESECTION

ER complications such as perforation and bleeding during ER can occur not only in beginners but also in experienced practitioners. Therefore, it is crucial to become familiar with the management of possible complications in ESD. This is because, in addition to complete resection, patient safety should always be considered during the ESD process.

1. Bleeding
   Endoscopic treatment for bleeding is essential during the resection process, as the occurrence of bleeding can worsen visibility and make the procedure very difficult. Even a small amount of bleeding can accumulate from multiple points,

making it difficult to secure a clear view or perform delicate hemostasis due to bloody staining of the submucosal layer. Therefore, it is advisable to perform hemostasis with hemostatic devices as much as possible whenever bleeding occurs and then proceed to the next step.

During the procedure, it is good to perform preventive hemostasis on the visible blood vessels before cutting them. When encountering thinner blood vessels during submucosal dissection, coagulation of vessels can be performed using the ESD knife by applying coagulation current at a lower current density than used for dissection. This can be achieved by placing more of the surface area of the knife on the vessel or decreasing the power setting on the ESU. However, for thicker, pulsating blood vessels, it is important to use coagulation graspers, using a pure coagulation current, to perform safe preventive coagulation. Occasionally, large pulsatile bleeding may occur during the cutting and submucosal dissection process, which should also be treated with coagulation graspers. Coagulation graspers are effective because they mechanically stop the flow of blood in vessels (preventing a heat sink effect by active blood flow) and by lowering the current density to effectively coagulate the blood vessel. If the use of coagulation graspers fails, consider using a hemostatic clip. Hemostatic clips can physically obstruct the cutting plane during ESD, so it is better to consider them as a last resort for massive bleeding that cannot be stopped by other methods. Careful treatment of exposed blood vessels after dissection completion can help prevent delayed bleeding. However, excessive coagulation during hemostasis should be avoided, as it can increase the risk of delayed perforation by damaging the muscle layer. Delayed Bleeding can occur after the ESD procedure, typically within the first few days. It can often be managed with endoscopic hemostasis or supportive care, such as blood transfusion if necessary.

2. Perforation

To prevent perforation, it is important to secure an adequate submucosal fluid cushion and to only cut or dissect when the knife tip can be visualized. Perforation can occur when operating blindly with an electronic knife, when making long continuous incisions, or when using a tip-shaped knife such as a needle knife or dual knife and the cutting direction is mistakenly directed toward the deeper layers. When using a knife, it is necessary to adhere to the principle of cutting while directly observing the knife tip, and when using a non-insulated cutting knife, it is important to operate the knife in a direction away from the muscle layer to prevent perforation. Performing the procedure while observing the cutting surface being dissected allows for a relatively safe dissection.

If a perforation occurs, in most cases, recovery is possible with endoscopic closure and conservative treatment. If a perforation occurs, minimize insufflation of gas to avoid expanding the perforation site and apply a clip to close the defect. It is preferable to quickly add dissection around the perforation site to secure space so that dissection can continue after closure of the perforation. If the perforation site is difficult to close with a clip, it is recommended to suture using a suture device such as an overstitch/T-tag. This procedure must be performed while thoroughly monitoring for signs of tension pneumoperitoneum, as excessive leakage of gas into the abdominal cavity due to perforation can compress the diaphragm upward, leading to respiratory distress. If the patient exhibits decreased oxygen saturation, it is necessary to quickly decompress by inserting an 18-gauge angiocatheter or Veress needle into the abdomen to decompress the peritoneum. Because gas rises to the right side of the abdomen in the left lateral position, puncturing the right 9 to 10 or 10 to 11 intercostal space and the intersection with the right midaxillary line can safely release the accumulated air above the liver. In the supine position, air can be released by puncturing the site where abdominal paracentesis is performed in the left lower abdomen.

3. Incomplete resection

   In some cases, ESD may not completely remove the lesion, leading to the possibility of residual or recurrent disease. Incomplete resection may be due to technical challenges, submucosal fibrosis, or a poorly delineated margin. If incomplete resection is identified during the procedure, additional dissection or a second resection attempt may be performed to ensure complete removal of the lesion. In some cases, close surveillance or additional treatment modalities, such as ablation or surgery, may be necessary.

4. Infection

   Infection is a rare but potential complication after ESD, which can manifest as fever, abdominal pain, and/or leukocytosis. Infection after ESD can be caused by factors such as perforation, contamination, poor wound healing, immunosuppression, and bacterial translocation. In some cases, prophylactic antibiotics may be administered to reduce the risk of infection. For example, in the case of ER procedure for dialysis patients, including those on hemodialysis and peritoneal dialysis, the use of prophylactic antibiotics may be recommended to reduce the risk of infection.

5. Stricture formation

   Strictures or stenosis may develop after ESD, particularly in cases where a large portion of the circumference of the GI tract (specially, esophagus, cardia, pylorus, ileocecal [IC] valve, anus, and so forth) is resected. Endoscopic balloon dilation or stent placement can be used to manage strictures.

6. Deep vein thrombosis (DVT) or pulmonary embolism (PE)

   Prolonged immobilization during or after the procedure may increase the risk of DVT or PE. Prophylactic anticoagulation and early mobilization may help reduce this risk in high-risk patients.

To minimize the risk of adverse events during ESD, it is crucial to ensure proper patient selection, have a well-trained and experienced endoscopist, and follow meticulous procedural techniques. Moreover, close postoperative monitoring and prompt management of complications are essential for a successful outcome.

CLINICAL MANAGEMENT AFTER ENDOSCOPIC RESECTION
Post-Endoscopic Submucosal Dissection Care for the Upper Gastrointestinal Tract

Following ESD for the esophagus, stomach, and duodenum, patients are recommended to fast for a certain amount of time to check for any potential complications before gradually introducing clear liquids and progressing to a soft diet as tolerated. Acid suppression therapy, such as proton-pump inhibitors (PPIs) or histamine H2-receptor antagonists, is essential for these areas. Stricture prevention measures, such as balloon dilation or steroid injection, may be needed for the esophagus, whereas prophylactic antibiotics can be considered for the stomach and duodenum when the risk of infection is high. Regular follow-up endoscopies are necessary to monitor for complications and recurrence.

Following gastric ESD, acid suppression therapy is essential for promoting the healing of artificial ulcers and preventing complications such as bleeding, stricture formation, and perforation. PPIs are the preferred choice for acid suppression therapy following ESD for esophageal and gastric lesions due to their superior efficacy in promoting ulcer healing and preventing complications. However, H2 blockers may be considered in cases where PPIs are contraindicated or not tolerated.

The recommended usage of PPI varies depending on the individual patient and the extent of the procedure. A general guideline is as follows:

- Initiate PPI therapy immediately after ESD.
- Administer PPIs once or twice daily at standard or double the standard dose, depending on the severity of the lesion and the risk of complications.
- Continue PPI treatment for 4 to 8 weeks, depending on the ulcer size and the patient's response to therapy.

H pylori infection is a known risk factor for gastric cancer, and eradication of the bacteria is essential for preventing recurrence and improving long-term outcomes post-ESD. The treatment should be tailored to the individual patient, considering local antibiotic resistance patterns and the patient's prior exposure to antibiotics. A general approach is as follows.

- Test for H pylori infection before ESD or during the post-ESD follow-up period, using methods such as histology, rapid urease test, urea breath test, or stool antigen test.
- If H pylori infection is confirmed, initiate eradication therapy. The choice of regimen depends on local antibiotic resistance patterns and patient factors. A common first-line treatment is a 10 to 14 day course of triple therapy, including a PPI, clarithromycin, and amoxicillin or metronidazole.
- After completing eradication therapy, confirm the success of treatment with a noninvasive test, such as the urea breath test or stool antigen test, typically 4 to 6 weeks after therapy.

Post-Endoscopic Submucosal Dissection Care for the Colon

After ESD for the colon, patients should fast for a certain amount time, and then gradually introduce clear liquids and transition to a low-residue diet once tolerated. Prophylactic antibiotics can be considered in cases with a high risk of infection.

ENDOSCOPIC RESECTION OUTCOMES
Esophagus

ER has become a standard treatment for early esophageal cancer, including early-stage squamous cell carcinoma and Barrett's esophagus-associated neoplasia, with ESD providing better outcomes for larger lesions and reduced recurrence rates compared with EMR.

1. Efficacy: ESD has demonstrated en bloc resection rates of 95.1% to 100% and curative resection rates of 88% to 89.4% for early esophageal cancer.[19–21]
2. Safety: The overall complication rate for esophageal ESD ranges between 5% and 15%, with bleeding (2.1%), perforation (5.0%), and stricture formation (11.6%) being the most common adverse events.[20,21]
3. Long-term outcomes: Studies have reported 5-year overall survival rates of 86.4% and disease-specific survival rates of 97.5% for early esophageal cancer treated with ESD.[22]

Stomach

ER has emerged as a standard treatment for EGC without lymph node metastasis, providing comparable survival rates and reduced morbidity compared with surgery.

ESD has been reported to achieve higher *en bloc* and curative resection rates than EMR, especially for larger lesions.[23]

1. Efficacy: ESD has demonstrated *en bloc* resection rates of 85% to 97% and curative resection rates of 71% to 82%.[24]
2. Safety: The overall complication rate for ESD/EMR ranges between 5% and 10%, with bleeding(9.3%/8.6%, including delayed bleeding) and perforation(4%/0.8%) being the most common adverse events.[23]
3. Long-term outcomes: Studies have reported 5-year overall survival rates of 96% and disease-specific survival rates of 99.4% for EGC treated with ESD.[25]

Colon

ER, particularly ESD, has gained recognition as a viable treatment option for early-stage colorectal cancer and large premalignant lesions, offering high curative resection rates and lower recurrence rates compared to EMR.[26]

1. Efficacy: ESD has achieved *en bloc* resection rates of 65% to 100% and R0 resection rates of 53% to 100% for early colorectal cancer and large adenomas.[27]
2. Safety: The complication rate for colorectal ESD varies, with the most common adverse events being bleeding (occurring in approximately 2.4%–5% of cases), perforation (found in around 4%–8% of cases), and recurrence rate (ranging between 1% and 3%).[28]
3. Long-term outcomes: Research has shown that early colorectal cancer treated with ESD has a 5-year overall survival rate of 92.3% and a disease-free survival rate of 99.6%.[29]

ER techniques, such as EMR and ESD, have shown promising results in treating early-stage stomach, colon, and esophageal cancers. Although outcomes may vary slightly between countries and institutions, these techniques continue to demonstrate significant potential. Furthermore, as endoscopic techniques and skills continue to advance, recent studies and analyses are revealing even better outcomes in the field, showcasing the ongoing progress in this area. High *en bloc* and curative resection rates, manageable complication rates, and favorable long-term survival rates showcase the potential of these minimally invasive approaches in the management of GI cancers. As ER techniques continue to advance and become more refined, they are expected to play an increasingly important role in the management of these malignancies. Ongoing research and development of novel endoscopic tools, as well as improvements in training and standardization of ER procedures, will be crucial in further optimizing patient outcomes and expanding the indications for ER in the treatment of GI malignancies.

THE FUTURE OF ENDOSCOPIC RESECTION FOR EARLY LUMINAL CANCER

As endoscopy continues to evolve, technological advancements in robotic assistance and innovative endoscopic tools are being developed, holding the potential to revolutionize ER by enhancing the accuracy, safety, and efficiency of these procedures, ultimately improving patient outcomes and expanding the range of treatable lesions.

Robotic assistance in ER can potentially improve the precision and safety of procedures by offering enhanced dexterity, improved visualization, and increased stability. For instance, the robotic-assisted ESD system enables the precise resection of lesions located in challenging anatomic sites, such as the colon or the esophagus, while minimizing the risk of complications. This technology can also reduce the physical strain on endoscopists, allowing for longer and more complex procedures. Innovative endoscopic tools, such as electrocautery knives, submucosal injection solutions, and endoscopic suturing, and closure devices, can also significantly impact the efficacy and safety of ER. For instance, novel electrocautery knives can improve cutting efficiency and reduce thermal damage to surrounding tissues, whereas advanced endoscopic suturing and closure devices can promote faster healing and minimize the risk of postprocedure complications. Moreover, the development of artificial intelligence (AI) and machine learning (ML) algorithms holds promise in enhancing the accuracy and efficiency of endoscopic procedures. For instance, AI-aided detection and characterization of colorectal polyps have shown high accuracy and could potentially reduce the need for unnecessary biopsies or surgeries.

In conclusion, the continuous development of technology in endoscopy offers the potential to revolutionize ER by improving accuracy, safety, and efficiency, leading to better patient outcomes and expanding the range of treatable lesions.

SUMMARY

"The Endoscopic Oncologist" refers to a medical professional who specializes in the ER of early luminal cancer. ER is a minimally invasive technique that involves the removal of early-stage tumors from the lining of the digestive tract.

ER is an effective and safe treatment option for early luminal cancer, which is cancer that is confined to the inner lining of the digestive tract. ER procedures can be performed using various techniques such as EMR or ESD. These techniques enable the removal of cancerous tissues while preserving the underlying layers of the digestive tract, thereby reducing the risk of complications such as bleeding, perforation, and stenosis.

The endoscopic oncologist is a highly skilled and specialized medical professional who is trained in the use of advanced endoscopic tools and techniques for the resection of early luminal cancer. The endoscopic oncologist works closely with a multidisciplinary team of health care professionals to ensure that patients receive comprehensive and personalized care.

Overall, the endoscopic oncologist plays a crucial role in the management of early luminal cancer, providing patients with a minimally invasive treatment option that offers excellent outcomes and a faster recovery time compared with traditional surgery.

DISCLOSURE

J.H. Hwang is a consultant for Boston Scientific, Olympus, Medtronic, FujiFILM, Lumendi, Neptune, and Micro-Tech. H.S. Choi has no disclosures.

CLINICS CARE POINTS

- Prior to performing endoscopic resection, the lesion should be evaluated carefully to confirm that the lesion is amenable to endoscopic resection. If there is any concern for advanced pathology, the case should be presented in a multidiciplinary conference prior to performing endoscopic resection.

- Patients undergoing endoscopic resection should be followed closely to monitor for any delayed complications such a bleeding or perforation.

- Following endoscopic resection, surveillance should be performed based on pathologic findings and established guidelines.

REFERENCES

1. Suzuki H, Oda I, Abe S, et al. High rate of 5-year survival among patients with early gastric cancer undergoing curative endoscopic submucosal dissection. Gastric Cancer 2016;19(1):198–205.
2. Moghimi-Dehkordi B, Safaee A. An overview of colorectal cancer survival rates and prognosis in Asia. World J Gastrointest Oncol 2012;4(4):71–5.
3. Gelberg HB. Comparative anatomy, physiology, and mechanisms of disease production of the esophagus, stomach, and small intestine. Toxicol Pathol 2014; 42(1):54–66.
4. Soybel DI. Anatomy and physiology of the stomach. Surg Clin North Am 2005; 85(5):875–94, v.
5. Sadalla S, Lisotti A, Fuccio L, et al. Colonoscopy-related colonic ischemia. World J Gastroenterol 2021;27(42):7299–310.
6. Torre LA, Siegel RL, Ward EM, et al. Global Cancer Incidence and Mortality Rates and Trends–An Update. Cancer Epidemiol Biomarkers Prev 2016;25(1):16–27.
7. Endoscopic Classification Review G. Update on the Paris classification of superficial neoplastic lesions in the digestive tract. Endoscopy 2005;37(6):570–8.
8. Draganov PV, Wang AY, Othman MO, et al. AGA Institute Clinical Practice Update: Endoscopic Submucosal Dissection in the United States. Clin Gastroenterol Hepatol 2019;17(1):16–25 e1.
9. Ishihara R, Arima M, Iizuka T, et al. Endoscopic submucosal dissection/endoscopic mucosal resection guidelines for esophageal cancer. Dig Endosc 2020; 32(4):452–93.
10. Gotoda T, Yanagisawa A, Sasako M, et al. Incidence of lymph node metastasis from early gastric cancer: estimation with a large number of cases at two large centers. Gastric Cancer 2000;3(4):219–25.
11. Shaukat A, Kaltenbach T, Dominitz JA, et al. Endoscopic Recognition and Management Strategies for Malignant Colorectal Polyps: Recommendations of the US Multi-Society Task Force on Colorectal Cancer. Gastrointest Endosc 2020; 92(5):997–1015 e1.
12. Committee AT, Maple JT, Abu Dayyeh BK, et al. Endoscopic submucosal dissection. Gastrointest Endosc 2015;81(6):1311–25.
13. Choi HS, Chun HJ. Accessory Devices Frequently Used for Endoscopic Submucosal Dissection. Clin Endosc 2017;50(3):224–33.
14. Maehata T, Goto O, Takeuchi H, et al. Cutting edge of endoscopic full-thickness resection for gastric tumor. World J Gastrointest Endosc 2015;7(16):1208–15.
15. Standards of Practice C, Faulx AL, Kothari S, et al. The role of endoscopy in subepithelial lesions of the GI tract. Gastrointest Endosc 2017;85(6):1117–32.
16. Hu JW, Zhang C, Chen T, et al. Submucosal tunneling endoscopic resection for the treatment of rectal submucosal tumors originating from the muscular propria layer. J Cancer Res Ther 2014;10(Suppl):281–6.
17. Cao B, Lu J, Tan Y, et al. Efficacy and safety of submucosal tunneling endoscopic resection for gastric submucosal tumors: a systematic review and meta-analysis. Rev Esp Enferm Dig 2021;113(1):52–9.
18. Choi HS, Chun HJ, Seo MH, et al. Endoscopic submucosal tunnel dissection salvage technique for ulcerative early gastric cancer. World J Gastroenterol 2014;20(27):9210–4.
19. Tsujii Y, Nishida T, Nishiyama O, et al. Clinical outcomes of endoscopic submucosal dissection for superficial esophageal neoplasms: a multicenter retrospective cohort study. Endoscopy 2015;47(9):775–83.

20. Ono S, Fujishiro M, Niimi K, et al. Long-term outcomes of endoscopic submucosal dissection for superficial esophageal squamous cell neoplasms. Gastrointest Endosc 2009;70(5):860–6.
21. Kim JS, Kim BW, Shin IS. Efficacy and safety of endoscopic submucosal dissection for superficial squamous esophageal neoplasia: a meta-analysis. Dig Dis Sci 2014;59(8):1862–9.
22. Yeh JH, Huang RY, Lee CT, et al. Long-term outcomes of endoscopic submucosal dissection and comparison to surgery for superficial esophageal squamous cancer: a systematic review and meta-analysis. Therap Adv Gastroenterol 2020;13. 1756284820964316.
23. Lian J, Chen S, Zhang Y, et al. A meta-analysis of endoscopic submucosal dissection and EMR for early gastric cancer. Gastrointest Endosc 2012;76(4): 763–70.
24. Daoud DC, Suter N, Durand M, et al. Comparing outcomes for endoscopic submucosal dissection between Eastern and Western countries: A systematic review and meta-analysis. World J Gastroenterol 2018;24(23):2518–36.
25. Abdelfatah MM, Barakat M, Ahmad D, et al. Long-term outcomes of endoscopic submucosal dissection versus surgery in early gastric cancer: a systematic review and meta-analysis. Eur J Gastroenterol Hepatol 2019;31(4):418–24.
26. Fujiya M, Tanaka K, Dokoshi T, et al. Efficacy and adverse events of EMR and endoscopic submucosal dissection for the treatment of colon neoplasms: a meta-analysis of studies comparing EMR and endoscopic submucosal dissection. Gastrointest Endosc 2015;81(3):583–95.
27. Repici A, Hassan C, De Paula Pessoa D, et al. Efficacy and safety of endoscopic submucosal dissection for colorectal neoplasia: a systematic review. Endoscopy 2012;44(2):137–50.
28. Lim XC, Nistala KRY, Ng CH, et al. Endoscopic submucosal dissection vs endoscopic mucosal resection for colorectal polyps: A meta-analysis and meta-regression with single arm analysis. World J Gastroenterol 2021;27(25):3925–39.
29. Boda K, Oka S, Tanaka S, et al. Clinical outcomes of endoscopic submucosal dissection for colorectal tumors: a large multicenter retrospective study from the Hiroshima GI Endoscopy Research Group. Gastrointest Endosc 2018;87(3): 714–22.

Endoscopic Ultrasound-Guided Antitumor Therapy

Yousuke Nakai, MD, PhD[a,b,*]

KEYWORDS

- Ablation • Fine-needle injection • Oncolytic viral therapy • Radiofrequency ablation
- Endoscopic ultrasound

KEY POINTS

- Various endoscopic ultrasound (EUS)-guided antitumor therapies such as injection, ablation, and radioactive seeds have been developed since its first clinical introduction in 2000.
- Both pancreatic solid tumors (carcinoma and neuroendocrine tumor) and cystic tumors are potential targets of EUS-guided treatment.
- The feasibility of EUS-guided antitumor therapy is established but randomized controlled trials are mandatory to confirm its role.
- In planning confirmatory clinical trials, we need to examine the goal of EUS-guided antitumor therapy, that is, definitive treatment for neuroendocrine neoplasms and adjunctive or immunomodulatory treatment of pancreatic cancer.

INTRODUCTION

Endoscopic ultrasound (EUS) was first developed as an imaging modality, but the real-time visualization of the needle by a linear-array echoendoscope allows EUS-guided fine-needle aspiration (EUS-FNA) for the pathologic diagnosis of variouslesions.[1,2] More recently, EUS has become more of a therapeutic procedure rather than just a diagnostic one. EUS-guided interventions started as drainage, access, and anastomosis[3] but have been investigated as antitumor therapy too.[4,5] Although any organ can be a treatment target, pancreatic cancer or its precursors have drawn major attention due to its dismal prognosis as well as easy access to the pancreas by EUS. In this article, the author discusses the role of EUS-guided antitumor therapy mainly for pancreatic tumors.

---

[a] Department of Gastroenterology, Graduate School of Medicine, The University of Tokyo, Tokyo, Japan; [b] Department of Endoscopy and Endoscopic Surgery, The University of Tokyo Hospital, 7-3-1 Hongo, Bunkyo-ku, Tokyo 113-8655, Japan
* Department of Endoscopy and Endoscopic Surgery, The University of Tokyo Hospital, 7-3-1 Hongo, Bunkyo-ku, Tokyo 113-8655, Japan.
E-mail address: ynakai-tky@umin.ac.jp

Gastrointest Endoscopy Clin N Am 34 (2024) 79–89
https://doi.org/10.1016/j.giec.2023.08.004
1052-5157/24/© 2023 Elsevier Inc. All rights reserved.

ENDOSCOPIC ULTRASOUND-GUIDED FINE-NEEDLE INJECTION FOR PANCREATIC SOLID TUMORS

EUS-guided fine-needle injection (EUS-FNI) is a delivery of various antitumor agents through the FNA needle under EUS guidance, and EUS-guided celiac plexus/ganglion neurolysis is the most clinically used procedure using EUS-FNI. The first trial of EUS-FNI as antitumor therapy for pancreatic cancer using cytoimplant was reported by Chang and colleagues in 2000.[6] Injection of cytoimplant, allogenic mixed lymphocyte culture, causes cytokine production directly within a tumor and can induce its regression by host antitumor effector mechanisms, in addition to the release of cytokines and the activation of immune effector cells. Because this study demonstrated safety and feasibility of EUS-FNI, various agents have been investigated as EUS-FNI for pancreatic cancer (**Table 1**). EUS-FNI can be classified as immunotherapy including cytoimplant, viral therapy, chemotherapy, and others. The largest clinical trial of EUS-FNI thus far was a randomized controlled trial of TNFerade biologic.[7] TNFerade biologic was constructed as a second-generation adenovector, which expresses the cDNA encoding human tumor necrosis factor (TNF). To further optimize local effectiveness and minimize systemic toxicity, the radiation-inducible immediate response Egr-1 (early growth response) promoter was placed upstream of the transcriptional start site of the human TNF contemporary deoxyribonucleic acid (cDNA). This vector was engineered to ensure that maximal gene expression and subsequent TNF secretion are constrained in space and time by radiation therapy. Thus, the trial was designed as a phase III trial comparing TNFerade biologic in combination with fluorouracil-based chemoradiation and fluorouracil-based chemoradiation alone, and a total of 304 patients with locally advanced pancreatic cancer were enrolled in the trial. The study failed to demonstrate superiority of additional EUS-FNI compared with the standard of care alone; the median overall survival was 10.0 months in both arms.

The negative results of this large phase III trial caused debate against the use of EUS-FNI as local treatment of the "systemic disease" of pancreatic cancer. However, the author has seen resurgence of various EUS-FNI studies recently using new agents such as STNM01[8] and Ad5-yCD/mutTK(SR39)rep-ADP (Ad5-DS).[9] STNM01 is a synthetic double-stranded RNA oligonucleotide designed to suppress carbohydrate sulfotransferase 15 gene expression through an RNA interference mechanism, which leads to inhibition of tumor growth as well as reduction in fibrosis. Ad5-DS is a second-generation replication-competent oncolytic adenovirus, which works as double-suicide gene therapy through conversion to 5-fluorouracil and valganciclovir-5-monophosphate. In these studies, EUS-FNI was performed in combination with systemic chemotherapy by S-1 or gemcitabine.

There are some possible explanations for this resurgence of EUS-FNI for pancreatic cancer: development of new chemotherapeutic regimens in pancreatic cancer and immunotherapy.[10] The development of new chemotherapeutic regimens such as FOLFIRINOX and nab-paclitaxel plus gemcitabine prolonged survival of advanced pancreatic cancer and made the treatment window period of EUS-FNI longer than before. In addition, immunotherapy such as programmed death receptor-1 (PD-1) and programmed death-ligand 1 (PD-L1) inhibitors provided better progression-free survival and overall survival in various cancers.[11] Those agents are effective in "immune hot" cancers but pancreatic cancer is known as "immune cold" cancer.[12] Local therapy, including EUS-FNI or ablation discussed below, can theoretically turn immune cold pancreatic cancer to immune hot. Thus, further investigation of direct antitumor and immune modulative effect of EUS-FNI is necessary. In a recent phase I/IIa trial of STNM01,[13] sequential EUS-FNA specimen during repeated EUS-FNI treatment

Table 1
Endoscopic ultrasound-guided fine-needle injection for pancreatic cancer

Author, Year	FNI Agent	Treatment Type	Study Design	n	Disease Extension	Response	Adverse Events	Survival (months)
Chang et al,[6] 2000	Cytoimplant	Immunotherapy	Phase 1	8	Unresectable	Partial remission 25%, minor response 12.5%	Fever	13.2
Hecht et al,[18] 2003	ONYX-015	Viral therapy	Phase 1/2	21	Unresectable	Partial response 10%	Perforation, sepsis	7.5
Irisawa et al,[19] 2007	Dendritic cells	Immunotherapy	Pilot	7	Unresectable	Minor response 28.6%	No	9
Hirooka et al,[20] 2009	Dendritic cells (OK-432 pulsed)	Immunotherapy	Phase 1	5	Locally advanced	Partial remission 20%	Anemia, leukocytopenia, constipation, nausea	15.9
Endo et al,[21] 2012	Dendritic cells (OK-432)	Immunotherapy	Phase 1	9	Resectable	Not available	Fever, pain, vomit, elevated liver enzymes	18
Hanna et al,[22] 2012	BC-819	Plasmid	Pilot	6	Unresectable	Partial response 33.3%	Diarrhea, fatigue, lipase elevation	—
Hecht et al,[23] 2012	TNFerade	Viral therapy	Phase 1/2	50	Locally advanced	Complete response 2%, partial response 6%, minor response 8%	Bleeding thrombosis, pain, pancreatitis	9.8
Herman et al,[7] 2013	TNFerade	Viral therapy	Phase 3	187	Locally advanced	Partial response 8.2%	nausea, pain, anorexia	10.0
Hirooka et al,[24] 2017	Dendritic cells (zoledronate-pulsed)	Immunotherapy	Phase 1/2	15	Locally advanced	No response, stable disease 46.7%	Fever	11.5
Levy et al,[25] 2017	Gemcitabine	Chemotherapy	Prospective	36	Unresectable	Partial response 25%	No	10.4
Hirooka et al,[26] 2018	HF-10	Viral therapy	Phase 1	12	Locally advanced	Partial response 25%	Perforation, liver dysfunction, neutropenia	5.5
Nishimura et al,[8] 2018	STNM01	Oligonucleotide	Pilot	6	Unresectable	NA	No	5.8

(continued on next page)

Table 1
(continued)

Author, Year	FNI Agent	Treatment Type	Study Design	n	Disease Extension	Response	Adverse Events	Survival (months)
Lee et al,[9] 2020	Ad5-DS	Viral therapy	Phase 1	9	Locally advanced	Partial response 11%	Fever, sweat	NA
Fujisawa et al,[13] 2022	STNM01	Oligonucleotide	Phase 1/2a	22	Unresectable	Complete response 4.5%, partial response 4.5%	Appetite loss, nausea, hyperamylasemia, leukocytopenia	7.8

showed the increase of tumor-infiltrating CD3+T cells at week 4 was associated with longer survival, suggesting the role of immune effects by EUS-FNI. However, it is unclear whether this change was evoked by EUS-FNI itself or not. Measurement methodology of immunomodulatory effect is another hurdle in EUS-FNI, which needs to be established and standardized.

Another indication of EUS-FNI for pancreatic solid tumors is ethanol ablation for pancreatic neuroendocrine neoplasms (pNENs).[14] As opposed to the aggressive nature of pancreatic cancer, the clinical course of pNEN is more indolent. Surgical resection is the standard of care for pNEN as it can grow and metastasize especially when the size is larger than 2 cm. Given the indolent nature of pNEN and invasiveness of pancreatic surgery, less invasive treatment is ideal in elderly patients with comorbidities. EUS-guided ethanol ablation for symptomatic pNEN was first reported by Jürgensen.[15] Repeated episodes of hypoglycemia due to insulinoma were managed by EUS-guided ethanol ablation, though the procedure was complicated by mild post-procedure pancreatitis. A recent systematic review of EUS-guided ethanol ablation for pNEN[16] revealed a technical success rate of 96.7% and a clinical success rate of 82.2%. The adverse event rate was 11.5%, and pancreatitis was the most common (7.6%) adverse event. In a meta-regression analysis, higher amount of ethanol injection was associated with adverse events. Thus, the appropriate amount of ethanol according to the size of pNEN should be further investigated. Pancreatic surgery is sometimes complicated by postoperative adverse events and might be too invasive for nonaggressive pNEN. In a propensity score-matched study in cases with small (<2 cm) pNEN,[17] EUS-guided ethanol ablation was associated with less early major adverse events (0% and 11.2%) and shorter hospital stay (4 and 14.1 days) compared with surgery. In terms of long-term outcomes, the overall and disease-specific survival was comparable between EUS-guided ethanol ablation and surgery. Thus, for small pNEN, EUS-guided ethanol ablation can be a treatment option, especially in elderly patients unfit for surgery.

RADIOFREQUENCY ABLATION AND OTHER ABLATIVE THERAPY

EUS-guided radiofrequency ablation (EUS-RFA) is another EUS-guided technique for tumor ablation. Percutaneous RFA has replaced ethanol ablation and has long been used for liver tumors.[27] The development of dedicated devices for EUS-RFA has allowed this technology to be used for pancreatic tumors,[28] and the feasibility of EUS-RFA for pNEN was reported in 2015.[29] In a systematic review, technical success rate (94.4%), clinical success rate (85.2%), and adverse event rate (14.1%) were comparable with EUS-guided ethanol ablation.[16] Similar to EUS-guided ethanol ablation, a propensity score-matched study in cases with insulinoma was recently reported comparing EUS-RFA and surgery.[30] Clinical efficacy was 95.5% for EUS-RFA compared with 100% in surgery, with a shorter hospital stay (3.4 and 11.1 days). Adverse event rates were 18% and 61.8%, respectively, and severe adverse events were only encountered after surgery (15.7%). Recurrence was more often seen after EUS-RFA, but 11 out of 15 recurrences after EUS-RFA were managed by another session of EUS-RFA. Thus, both EUS-ethanol ablation and EUS-RFA can be a first-line treatment option for pNEN, but randomized controlled trials are necessary to confirm its role in surgically fit patients. Furthermore, treatment selection between EUS-guided ablation and surgery would be more important in the era of less invasive laparoscopic or robotic pancreatic surgery.

EUS-RFA for advanced pancreatic cancer has been attempted too, but its role is even more unclear at this point. Pilot studies of EUS-RFA demonstrated safety and feasibility in pancreatic cancer.[31–33] A recent prospective study revealed promising long-term outcomes of EUS-RFA in combination with systemic chemotherapy with a median overall survival of 20 to 24 months in locally advanced or metastatic pancreatic cancer.[34] EUS-guided photodynamic therapy (EUS-PDT) is another treatment option. PDT enables specific ablation of tumor using a photosensitizer in combination with light irradiation. The feasibility of EUS-PDT for pancreatobiliary malignancy has been reported with acceptable safety in a few studies.[35–37] Future research should focus on the standardization of EUS-RFA/PDT in terms of indications (tumor extension, the first line or refractory, and so forth), the ablation setting, and the number of sessions as well as combination therapy using systemic chemotherapy regimens.

EUS-guided brachytherapy, the implantation of radioactive seeds under EUS-guidance, has also been reported for pancreatic cancer. EUS-guided fiducial marker placement for radiation therapy has long been used because of precise identification of pancreatic tumors as well as proximity to the stomach or duodenum by EUS.[38] Recently, dedicated EUS-guided fiducial markers have become commercially available.[39] As such, it is natural to use this technique for brachytherapy to treat pancreatic cancer. Most studies of EUS-guided brachytherapy were reported from China. Two pilot studies using [125]iodine seeds demonstrated response rates of 13.6% to 27%.[40,41] The feasibility of EUS-guided chemoradiation by intratumoral implants of both radioactive seeds and interstitial fluorouracil delivery was also feasible.[42] To further enhance antitumor effects of EUS-guided brachytherapy, a new computer-assisted treatment-planning system was developed.[43] In cases where the minimal peripheral dose was larger than 90 Gy, response rate was as high as 80%, suggesting the role of this new EUS-based treatment-planning system. A comparison of technical feasibility, safety, and efficacy between EUS-guided brachytherapy and new carbon ion or proton radiotherapy is mandatory to further increase its generalizability.

ENDOSCOPIC ULTRASOUND-GUIDED FINE-NEEDLE INJECTION FOR PANCREATIC CYSTIC NEOPLASMS

Pancreatic cystic neoplasms (PCNs) such as intraductal papillary mucinous neoplasms (IPMNs) and mucinous cystic neoplasms are well-known precursors of pancreatic cancer. Recommendations of diagnosis and surveillance for PCNs have been published, but the long-term cancer risk of PCNs necessitates lifelong surveillance, which poses physiologic, economic, and psychological burden to patients with PCNs. In addition to the low diagnostic yield of PCNs by the conventional modalities, the lack of interventions to prevent or reduce the risk of cancer is one of the major issues in the management of PCNs. In colorectal cancer, endoscopic surveillance and resection of adenomas can reduce the risk of and mortality by colorectal cancer, and chemoprevention has been investigated as well. In this context, EUS-guided ablation of PCNs was reported in 2005.[44] Thereafter, clinical trials of EUS-guided ablation of PCNs were published using chemotherapeutic agents such as paclitaxel and gemcitabine in addition to ethanol. A systematic review of EUS-guided ablation of PCNs revealed that the complete resolution rate was higher in paclitaxel-based regimens (63.6%) than in ethanol alone (32.8%). The adverse event rates were comparable between paclitaxel-based regimens (15%) and ethanol (21.2%).[45]

Despite these promising results, the indications of EUS-guided ablation are not well established. Although a Korean expert group excluded PCNs communicating with the pancreatic duct, that is, IPMNs, a US expert group included IPMNs as indications of EUS-guided ablation. A position statement by an international expert committee was published in 2019.[46] In this statement, indications for EUS-guided ablation are patients who are not surgical candidates or refuse surgery with a reasonable life expectancy; patients with a unilocular or oligolocular cyst with a presumed or confirmed diagnosis of a mucinous pancreatic cyst; and enlarging pancreatic cysts with a diameter of greater than 2 cm or pancreatic cysts with diameter of greater than 3 cm in size. On the other hand, the following characteristics are considered as relative contraindications: cyst with enhancing mural nodules, cyst with no or low malignant potential, dilated main pancreatic duct (MPD) > 5 mm in size, clear open communication of the cyst with the main pancreatic duct, more than 6 locules comprising the cyst, thick walls, thick septations, MPD stricture with pancreatic tail atrophy, significant solid components within the cyst, and a past medical history of acute pancreatitis.

Although there still remains controversy over its indications, the long-term outcomes of EUS-guided ablation of PCNs are promising.[47] A prospective study including 164 PCNs, of which 63 were indeterminate cysts, revealed that complete resolution rate was as high as 72.2% with a recurrence rate of only 1.7% during the median follow-up of 6 years. Although the abovementioned study results demonstrated long-term effectiveness of EUS-guided ablation of PCNs, malignant conversion after EUS-guided ablation of IPMN was reported too. In one case series study, two of eight cases had tumor spillage or dissemination at the time of surgery.[48] Furthermore, because IPMNs are felt to demonstrate two types of cancer progression, that is pancreatic cancer derived from IPMN and concomitant with IPMN,[49] it is questionable whether ablation of PCNs alone can actually reduce the risk of overall cancer progression. Furthermore, IPMNs are often multicentric and would need surveillance even after EUS-guided ablation. Therefore, there are still many unanswered questions such as indications, best agents for ablation, and the follow-up after ablation. The establishment of indications is mandatory to generalize this potentially useful procedure.

FUTURE PERSPECTIVE

As discussed above, EUS-guided antitumor therapy is based on the "delivery" of drugs, energy, or seeds for ablation and has sprouted various treatment options by using the advantage of precise tumor identification under EUS-guidance as well as the development of new devices. On the other hand, most studies reported so far were single-arm studies with a small sample size, and the lack of a control group was the major limitation. There have been no large-scale clinical trials of EUS-guided antitumor therapy because the only RCT of TNFerade failed to demonstrate the superiority of EUS-FNI.[7]

One of the recent developments of anticancer treatment is establishment of immunotherapy. Pancreatic cancer is well known as an "immune cold" cancer, but in addition to immunotherapy via EUS-FNI itself, local ablative treatment can theoretically evoke immune response and enhance immunotherapy too. In addition to the conventional tumor response evaluation such as RECIST, we need to establish methods to measure immune effects by EUS-guided local therapy, especially in combination with systemic chemotherapy.

Although various abovementioned modalities have been developed for EUS-guided antitumor therapy, high-quality evidence by head-to-head comparative studies is still lacking. In addition, the exact details of procedures are often endosonographer-dependent and different at each expert center. Standardization among experts is warranted before a multicenter comparative study is to be conducted.

Last but not least, the indication and goal of EUS-guided antitumor therapy should be established for each disease entity and treatment modality. For example, the indication of EUS-guided ablation for pNEN should be evaluated in comparison with radical surgical resection and the goal should be set as complete ablation with less adverse events. On the other hand, the indication of EUS-guided ablation for pancreatic cancer is palliative at this point, and the treatment goal might be the control of symptoms, tumor volume reduction, and/or immunomodulatory effects in combination with systemic chemotherapy. Finally, the indication of EUS-guided ablation for PCNs is still under debate, and the content and amount of injection are far from standardized. The goal should not be the resolution of PCNs because most of them are incidental and asymptomatic. The goal should be the long-term incidence of pancreatic cancer.

In summary, EUS-guided anticancer treatment holds promise in the recent era of development of new chemotherapy and immunotherapy for pancreatic tumors. However, the lack of large-scale data with a control group and standardization of procedures is major drawbacks. Thus, the collaboration of endosonographers with medical oncologists and surgeons is mandatory to further advance this promising but preliminary EUS-guided anticancer treatment into the standard of care management.

CLINICS CARE POINTS

- Endoscopic ultrasound (EUS)-guided antitumor therapy should be performed under a clinical trial protocol.
- Pancreatitis should be ruled out in cases with pain after EUS-guided antitumor therapy for pancreatic lesions.
- Long-term follow-up by imaging modalities such as computed tomography (CT) and EUS is necessary to confirm treatment responses.

DISCLOSURE

Y. Nakai received research grant from Fujifilm, Japan and HOYA Pentax and honoraria from Fujifilm.

REFERENCES

1. Vilmann P, Jacobsen GK, Henriksen FW, et al. Endoscopic ultrasonography with guided fine needle aspiration biopsy in pancreatic disease. Gastrointest Endosc 1992;38(2):172–3.
2. Chang KJ, Albers CG, Erickson RA, et al. Endoscopic ultrasound-guided fine needle aspiration of pancreatic carcinoma. Am J Gastroenterol 1994;89(2): 263–6.
3. Duarte-Chavez R, Kahaleh M. Therapeutic endoscopic ultrasound. Transl Gastroenterol Hepatol 2022;7:20.
4. Nakai Y, Chang KJ. Endoscopic ultrasound-guided antitumor agents. Gastrointestinal endoscopy clinics of North America 2012;22(2):315–24, x.
5. Han J, Chang KJ. Endoscopic Ultrasound-Guided Direct Intervention for Solid Pancreatic Tumors. Clinical endoscopy 2017;50(2):126–37.
6. Chang KJ, Nguyen PT, Thompson JA, et al. Phase I clinical trial of allogeneic mixed lymphocyte culture (cytoimplant) delivered by endoscopic ultrasound-guided fine-needle injection in patients with advanced pancreatic carcinoma. Cancer 2000;88(6):1325–35.

7. Herman JM, Wild AT, Wang H, et al. Randomized phase III multi-institutional study of TNFerade biologic with fluorouracil and radiotherapy for locally advanced pancreatic cancer: final results. J Clin Oncol 2013;31(7):886–94.

8. Nishimura M, Matsukawa M, Fujii Y, et al. Effects of EUS-guided intratumoral injection of oligonucleotide STNM01 on tumor growth, histology, and overall survival in patients with unresectable pancreatic cancer. Gastrointest Endosc 2018;87(4):1126–31.

9. Lee JC, Shin DW, Park H, et al. Tolerability and safety of EUS-injected adenovirus-mediated double-suicide gene therapy with chemotherapy in locally advanced pancreatic cancer: a phase 1 trial. Gastrointest Endosc 2020;92(5):1044–52.e1041.

10. Nakai Y, Chang KJ. EUS-guided fine-needle injection for pancreatic cancer: back to the future. Gastrointest Endosc 2020;92(5):1053–4.

11. Sharma P, Goswami S, Raychaudhuri D, et al. Immune checkpoint therapy-current perspectives and future directions. Cell 2023;186(8):1652–69.

12. Schumacher TN, Schreiber RD. Neoantigens in cancer immunotherapy. Science 2015;348(6230):69–74.

13. Fujisawa T, Tsuchiya T, Kato M, et al. STNM01, the RNA oligonucleotide targeting carbohydrate sulfotransferase 15, as second-line therapy for chemotherapy-refractory patients with unresectable pancreatic cancer: An open label, phase I/IIa trial. EClinicalMedicine 2023;55:101731.

14. Rimbaş M, Horumbă M, Rizzatti G, et al. Interventional endoscopic ultrasound for pancreatic neuroendocrine neoplasms. Dig Endosc 2020;32(7):1031–41.

15. Jürgensen C, Schuppan D, Neser F, et al. EUS-guided alcohol ablation of an insulinoma. Gastrointest Endosc 2006;63(7):1059–62.

16. Garg R, Mohammed A, Singh A, et al. EUS-guided radiofrequency and ethanol ablation for pancreatic neuroendocrine tumors: A systematic review and meta-analysis. Endoscopic ultrasound 2022;11(3):170–85.

17. So H, Ko SW, Shin SH, et al. Comparison of EUS-guided ablation and surgical resection for nonfunctioning small pancreatic neuroendocrine tumors: a propensity score-matching study. Gastrointest Endosc 2023;97(4):741–51.e741.

18. Hecht JR, Bedford R, Abbruzzese JL, et al. A phase I/II trial of intratumoral endoscopic ultrasound injection of ONYX-015 with intravenous gemcitabine in unresectable pancreatic carcinoma. Clin Cancer Res 2003;9(2):555–61.

19. Irisawa A, Takagi T, Kanazawa M, et al. Endoscopic ultrasound-guided fine-needle injection of immature dendritic cells into advanced pancreatic cancer refractory to gemcitabine: a pilot study. Pancreas 2007;35(2):189–90.

20. Hirooka Y, Itoh A, Kawashima H, et al. A combination therapy of gemcitabine with immunotherapy for patients with inoperable locally advanced pancreatic cancer. Pancreas 2009;38(3):e69–74.

21. Endo H, Saito T, Kenjo A, et al. Phase I trial of preoperative intratumoral injection of immature dendritic cells and OK-432 for resectable pancreatic cancer patients. J Hepato-Biliary-Pancreatic Sci 2012;19(4):465–75.

22. Hanna N, Ohana P, Konikoff FM, et al. Phase 1/2a, dose-escalation, safety, pharmacokinetic and preliminary efficacy study of intratumoral administration of BC-819 in patients with unresectable pancreatic cancer. Cancer Gene Ther 2012; 19(6):374–81.

23. Hecht JR, Farrell JJ, Senzer N, et al. EUS or percutaneously guided intratumoral TNFerade biologic with 5-fluorouracil and radiotherapy for first-line treatment of locally advanced pancreatic cancer: a phase I/II study. Gastrointest Endosc 2012;75(2):332–8.

24. Hirooka Y, Kawashima H, Ohno E, et al. Comprehensive immunotherapy combined with intratumoral injection of zoledronate-pulsed dendritic cells, intravenous adoptive activated T lymphocyte and gemcitabine in unresectable locally advanced pancreatic carcinoma: a phase I/II trial. Oncotarget 2018;9(2): 2838–47.

25. Levy MJ, Alberts SR, Bamlet WR, et al. EUS-guided fine-needle injection of gemcitabine for locally advanced and metastatic pancreatic cancer. Gastrointest Endosc 2017;86(1):161–9.

26. Hirooka Y, Kasuya H, Ishikawa T, et al. A Phase I clinical trial of EUS-guided intratumoral injection of the oncolytic virus, HF10 for unresectable locally advanced pancreatic cancer. BMC Cancer 2018;18(1):596.

27. Shiina S, Teratani T, Obi S, et al. A randomized controlled trial of radiofrequency ablation with ethanol injection for small hepatocellular carcinoma. Gastroenterology 2005;129(1):122–30.

28. Kim HJ, Seo DW, Hassanuddin A, et al. EUS-guided radiofrequency ablation of the porcine pancreas. Gastrointest Endosc 2012;76(5):1039–43.

29. Armellini E, Crinò SF, Ballarè M, et al. Endoscopic ultrasound-guided radiofrequency ablation of a pancreatic neuroendocrine tumor. Endoscopy 2015; 47(Suppl 1 UCTN):E600–1.

30. Crinò SF, Napoleon B, Facciorusso A, et al. Endoscopic Ultrasound-guided Radiofrequency Ablation Versus Surgical Resection for Treatment of Pancreatic Insulinoma. Clin Gastroenterol Hepatol 2023. https://doi.org/10.1016/j.cgh.2023. 02.022.

31. Lakhtakia S, Ramchandani M, Galasso D, et al. EUS-guided radiofrequency ablation for management of pancreatic insulinoma by using a novel needle electrode (with videos). Gastrointest Endosc 2016;83(1):234–9.

32. Song TJ, Seo DW, Lakhtakia S, et al. Initial experience of EUS-guided radiofrequency ablation of unresectable pancreatic cancer. Gastrointest Endosc 2016; 83(2):440–3.

33. Scopelliti F, Pea A, Conigliaro R, et al. Technique, safety, and feasibility of EUS-guided radiofrequency ablation in unresectable pancreatic cancer. Surg Endosc 2018;32(9):4022–8.

34. Oh D, Seo DW, Song TJ, et al. Clinical outcomes of EUS-guided radiofrequency ablation for unresectable pancreatic cancer: A prospective observational study. Endoscopic ultrasound 2022;11(1):68–74.

35. Choi JH, Oh D, Lee JH, et al. Initial human experience of endoscopic ultrasound-guided photodynamic therapy with a novel photosensitizer and a flexible laser-light catheter. Endoscopy 2015;47(11):1035–8.

36. DeWitt JM, Sandrasegaran K, O'Neil B, et al. Phase 1 study of EUS-guided photodynamic therapy for locally advanced pancreatic cancer. Gastrointest Endosc 2019;89(2):390–8.

37. Hanada Y, Pereira SP, Pogue B, et al. EUS-guided verteporfin photodynamic therapy for pancreatic cancer. Gastrointest Endosc 2021;94(1):179–86.

38. Park WG, Yan BM, Schellenberg D, et al. EUS-guided gold fiducial insertion for image-guided radiation therapy of pancreatic cancer: 50 successful cases without fluoroscopy. Gastrointest Endosc 2010;71(3):513–8.

39. Glissen Brown JR, Perumpail RB, Duran JF, et al. Preloaded 22-gauge fine-needle system facilitates placement of a higher number of fiducials for image-guided radiation therapy compared with traditional backloaded 19-gauge approach. Gastrointest Endosc 2021;94(5):953–8.

40. Sun S, Xu H, Xin J, et al. Endoscopic ultrasound-guided interstitial brachytherapy of unresectable pancreatic cancer: results of a pilot trial. Endoscopy 2006;38(4): 399–403.
41. Jin Z, Du Y, Li Z, et al. Endoscopic ultrasonography-guided interstitial implantation of iodine 125-seeds combined with chemotherapy in the treatment of unresectable pancreatic carcinoma: a prospective pilot study. Endoscopy 2008; 40(4):314–20.
42. Sun S, Ge N, Wang S, et al. Pilot trial of endoscopic ultrasound-guided interstitial chemoradiation of UICC-T4 pancreatic cancer. Endoscopic ultrasound 2012; 1(1):41–7.
43. Sun X, Lu Z, Wu Y, et al. An endoscopic ultrasonography-guided interstitial brachytherapy based special treatment-planning system for unresectable pancreatic cancer. Oncotarget 2017;8(45):79099–110.
44. Gan SI, Thompson CC, Lauwers GY, et al. Ethanol lavage of pancreatic cystic lesions: initial pilot study. Gastrointest Endosc 2005;61(6):746–52.
45. Attila T, Adsay V, Faigel DO. The efficacy and safety of endoscopic ultrasound-guided ablation of pancreatic cysts with alcohol and paclitaxel: a systematic review. Eur J Gastroenterol Hepatol 2019;31(1):1–9.
46. Teoh AY, Seo DW, Brugge W, et al. Position statement on EUS-guided ablation of pancreatic cystic neoplasms from an international expert panel. Endosc Int Open 2019;7(9):E1064–77.
47. Choi JH, Seo DW, Song TJ, et al. Long-term outcomes after endoscopic ultrasound-guided ablation of pancreatic cysts. Endoscopy 2017;49(9):866–73.
48. Jang JY, Byun Y, Han Y, et al. Malignant conversion and peritoneal dissemination after endoscopic ultrasound-guided ethanol ablation in intraductal papillary mucinous neoplasm of the pancreas. J Hepato-Biliary-Pancreatic Sci 2019; 26(10):467–72.
49. Oyama H, Tada M, Takagi K, et al. Long-term Risk of Malignancy in Branch-Duct Intraductal Papillary Mucinous Neoplasms. Gastroenterology 2020;158(1): 226–37.e225.

Endoscopic Palliative Therapies for Esophageal Cancer

Youssef Y. Soliman, MD[a], Madappa Kundranda, MD, PhD[b],
Toufic Kachaamy, MD[a],*

KEYWORDS

- Dysphagia • Quality of life • Palliation • Esophageal cancer • Esophageal stent
- Cryotherapy • Chemotherapy • Radiotherapy

KEY POINTS

- Palliation for patients with inoperable esophageal cancer involves local and systemic treatment modalities.
- Combinations of different modalities can improve outcomes but expose patients to more adverse events.
- For endoscopic treatments, severe dysphagia due to obstruction is best treated with stents, whereas mild-to-moderate dysphagia due to partial obstruction can be treated with ablative modalities.
- Data are emerging on intensive cryotherapy regimens and possible synergy with systemic therapy.

 Video content accompanies this article at http://www.giendo.theclinics.com.

INTRODUCTION

Esophageal cancer is the eighth most common cancer in the world, and the sixth leading cause of cancer death.[1] In the United States, approximately 20,000 new cases (the majority being adenocarcinoma), with 16,000 deaths, are identified on an annual basis.[2] The 5-year survival rate is about 20%. This in part is due to the late stage at diagnosis. Approximately 20% of patients present with localized disease. A third have locoregional disease (ie, with involvement of regional lymph nodes), and another 33% have distant metastases. The remaining 10% to 13% are not categorized.[3] In medically fit patients with localized and locoregional disease, the standard of care is

[a] Gastroenterology, City of Hope Phoenix, 14200 W Celebrate Life Way, Goodyear, AZ 85338, USA; [b] Gastrointestinal Oncology, Banner MD Anderson Cancer Center, Banner Gateway Medical Center, 2946 East Banner Gateway Drive, Gilbert, AZ 85324, USA
* Corresponding author. 14200 Celebrate Life Way, Goodyear, AZ 85338.
E-mail address: toufic.kachaamy@coh.org

Gastrointest Endoscopy Clin N Am 34 (2024) 91–110
https://doi.org/10.1016/j.giec.2023.07.003
1052-5157/24/© 2023 Elsevier Inc. All rights reserved.

neoadjuvant chemoradiation or chemotherapy followed by surgical resection and is associated with survival benefit.[4,5] However, despite advances in neoadjuvant treatments, up to 17% of potential surgical candidates do not undergo surgical resection because of disease progression or comorbidities.[6]

In patients who do not undergo surgical resection, dysphagia is the most common symptom. It may contribute to weight loss, malnutrition, and an overall decrease in quality of life (QOL).[7] Dysphagia most commonly develops due to obstruction by the esophageal mass. The National Comprehensive Cancer Network (NCCN) recommends interventions for palliation for patients with severe dysphagia while carefully weighing the benefits and risks of interventions in patients with mild-to-moderate dysphagia.[8] The objectives for palliation of obstruction in esophageal cancer are to improve dysphagia, disease specific QOL, and global QOL. The optimal strategy and modality are not established, and current practices are dependent on local expertise and patient preferences. They often involve a combination or sequence of multiple modalities of treatment and are best determined in a multidisciplinary way.

TREATMENT MODALITIES

To guide patients on the available endoscopic modalities for palliation, it is important for the endoscopist to be well versed with nonendoscopic modalities available, their benefits, adverse events, time to improvement and expected duration of effect. In addition, it is important to understand how endoscopic and nonendoscopic modalities can influence each other. It is also important to understand the heterogeneity of the outcomes studied. For instance, most studies evaluate dysphagia on a 5-point scale and quantify improvement by comparing scores preintervention and postintervention[9] (**Box 1**). Other studies evaluate improvement as dysphagia-free or the ability to swallow everything. More recently, studies evaluate dysphagia palliation in relation to QOL using global (EORTC-QOL30) and disease-specific (EORTC-QOL18) measures (**Box 2**).[10]

NONENDOSCOPIC MODALITIES FOR PALLIATION OF ESOPHAGEAL CANCER RELATED OBSTRUCTION

Multiple modalities exist for palliation of esophageal cancer. Surgical bypass and palliative esophagectomy are rarely considered due to unacceptable rates of morbidity and mortality.[11–14]

Box 1
Dysphagia scores on a 5-point scale. Most studies compare scores assigned preintervention and postintervention

Dysphagia
Scoring
Scale

0	Able to consume a normal diet
1	Dysphagia with certain solid foods
2	Able to swallow semisolid soft foods
3	Able to swallow liquids only
4	Unable to swallow saliva (complete dysphagia)

Adapted from Mellow MH, Pinkas H. Endoscopic therapy for esophageal carcinoma with Nd:YAG laser: prospective evaluation of efficacy, complications, and survival. Gastrointest Endosc. 1984;30(6):334-339. https://doi.org/10.1016/s0016-5107(8472448-5)

Box 2
Quality of life–driven score for patients with esophageal cancer

EORTC QLQ – OES18

Patients sometimes report that they have the following symptoms or problems. Please indicate the extent to which you have experienced these symptoms or problems <u>during the past week</u>. Please answer by circling the number that best applies to you.

During the past week:	Not at all	A little	Quite a bit	Very much
31. Could you eat solid food?	1	2	3	4
32. Could you eat liquidised or soft food?	1	2	3	4
33. Could you drink liquids?	1	2	3	4
34. Have you had trouble with swallowing your saliva?	1	2	3	4
35. Have you choked when swallowing?	1	2	3	4
36. Have you had trouble enjoying your meals?	1	2	3	4
37. Have you felt full up too quickly?	1	2	3	4
38. Have you had trouble with eating?	1	2	3	4
39. Have you had trouble with eating in front of other people?	1	2	3	4
40. Have you had a dry mouth?	1	2	3	4
41. Did food and drink taste different from usual?	1	2	3	4
42 Have you had trouble with coughing?	1	2	3	4
43. Have you had trouble with talking?	1	2	3	4
44. Have you had acid indigestion or heartburn?	1	2	3	4
45. Have you had trouble with acid or bile coming into your mouth?	1	2	3	4
46. Have you had pain when you eat?	1	2	3	4
47. Have you had pain in your chest?	1	2	3	4
48. Have you had pain in your stomach?	1	2	3	4

RADIATION THERAPY

Radiation therapy (RT) can be delivered by 2 different modalities: External beam radiotherapy (EBRT) or brachytherapy. In addition, RT can be used alone or in combination with other modalities such as chemotherapy, thermal/cryotherapy ablation, chemoradiation, or stenting in palliating dysphagia. EBRT uses an external source for radiation to target tissues. Modern EBRT can include three-dimensional conformal radiation therapy, intensity-modulated radiation therapy, volumetric modulated arc radiation therapy or Rapid Arc, image-guided radiation therapy, or stereotactic body radiation therapy. In general, it can take 2 to 8 weeks to experience improvement in dysphagia in ~70% of patients, with up to 30% initial worsening of symptoms before improvement.[15,16] Radiation-induced strictures occur in ~30% of cases at high doses. Approximately 40% of patients have symptom recurrence and require additional treatment modalities.[15,16] The balance of benefits and side effects has been correlated to differential dosing and frequency of EBRT, with trends of accelerated frequency[17] and lower cumulative doses (eg, total of 20 Gy VS 40+ Gy) being associated with comparable rates of, and time to, improvement with slightly lower need for interventions with other modalities (26% vs 40%).[18] This led most centers to adopt lower doses on an accelerated regimen as the preferred palliative modality. A recent review of the National Cancer Database cohort found that 1 out of 3 patients with stage IV esophageal cancer underwent EBRT without an associated survival advantage. Unfortunately, this database does not capture the indication for radiation and thus outcomes related to dysphagia and QOL could not be ascertained.[19]

BRACHYTHERAPY

Brachytherapy involves the precise placement of short-range radiation sources to deliver higher radiation doses to a target lesion while sparing surrounding tissue as possible. It entails endoscopic placement of a guiding catheter with a guidewire to identify the tumor. The radiation component needs to be done in the radiotherapy suite, where a radioactive intraluminal catheter is inserted to correspond to the desired margins of treatment.[20] This creates complexity in scheduling because either the patient will need to be transferred to the radiology department or the endoscopy equipment will need to have been set up in the radiation suite. Because of the ability to directly irradiate the tumor from the esophageal lumen, an overall lower dose of radiation can be used. This results in focused local radiation with high dose to the target lesion and less radiation to the surrounding tissues and structures.

Brachytherapy is contraindicated if the tumor extends into the trachea or bronchus due to the risk of fistulization and perforation. It is also contraindicated in the upper esophagus and in case of complete obstruction where the applicator cannot be placed. Brachytherapy has been studied prospectively and has been found to be effective in treating dysphagia with symptom resolution in 87% of patients after 1 month, 66% in 3 months, and 50% after 6 months.[21] Although effective, complications include fistulization (up to 34%), strictures (up to 42%), and esophagitis (up to 12.5%).[18] Two RCTs compared brachytherapy with stent placement.[22,23] Patients who received stents had faster improvement in dysphagia, although long-term QOL metrics favored brachytherapy. The complication rate was higher in the stent groups (33%) than in the brachytherapy group (21%), although both groups had a complication rate greater than 20%. There was no difference in survival.[22,23] The most recent systematic review on this topic found a rate of dysphagia improvement ranging from 50% to 100% with brachytherapy.[24] The complication rates, limited expertise, and complicated logistics (between endoscopy and radiation units) contribute to the relative limited use of a fairly effective modality.[25,26]

SYSTEMIC THERAPY

Systemic therapy is considered first-line therapy due to positive effects on survival in patients with inoperable esophageal cancer. This paradigm is rapidly evolving especially with the recent emergence of immunotherapy. The most recent Cochrane review[27] of 41 randomized control trials (RCTs) with 11,853 participants concluded that people who receive more agents (cytostatic or targeted therapies)—whether first-line or second-line treatments—have a survival advantage. The data on QOL in this review were limited mostly due to the low sample size and incompleteness of the data. One agent, ramucirumab, was found to be associated with a trend toward improved QOL for patients who received monotherapy after disease progression on first-line cytostatic treatments.[28] Specifically for esophageal cancer, 19 studies were included and reported survival outcomes in favor of systemic therapy. Concerning QOL outcomes, 11 studies showed no significant differences between systemic therapy and best supportive care and 8 studies showed improvement in QOL measures in patients receiving systemic therapy at the cost of increased toxicity. The most recent review on this topic found a significant gap in the impact of newer systemic agents including targeted and immunotherapy on symptoms and QOL outcomes due to the nature of data collected, which limits the ability to draw conclusions on efficacy on patient-centered outcomes.[29] Limited data exist on timing of improvement and amount of improvement in symptoms. From the available data, it seems that systemic therapy improves dysphagia in around half of the patients within a few weeks and this relief lasts around 1 to 2 months. A minority of patients will become dysphagia-free and have relief for up to 5 months.[30–32] The most recent Cochrane analysis on this topic recommended against using chemotherapy alone for long-term palliation of dysphagia because of the high rate of symptoms recurrence and the NCCN guidelines state that for long-term relief of dysphagia, an adjunct modality may be used in addition to systemic therapy.[8]

CHEMORADIOTHERAPY

An overall survival benefit with chemoradiation was demonstrated in a multicenter RCT of 368 patients by the CROSS group. In patients with resectable tumors, patients who underwent neoadjuvant concurrent chemoradiation for 5 weeks (weekly carboplatin and paclitaxel, and radiotherapy 5 d/wk) followed by surgery had a median survival of 49.4 months compared with 24 months in patients who underwent surgery alone.[33] However, for patients with inoperable esophageal cancer, compared with radiotherapy (30–35 Gy during 2–3 weeks) alone, the addition of chemotherapy (fluorouracil and cisplatin on days 1–4 of radiotherapy) did not show a compelling improvement in overall survival (6.7 vs 6.9 months) or dysphagia (3.4 vs 4.1 months) but had more grade 3 to 4 acute toxicity (36% vs 16%).[34] Therefore, for patients with stage IV disease, most centers that use radiation avoid concurrent fluorouracil and cisplatin-based chemotherapy.

ENDOSCOPIC MODALITIES
Laser Therapy

Neodymium-yttrium aluminum garnet (Nd:YAG) laser was introduced in the 1980s as a thermal modality for palliation of esophageal cancer.[35] Following thermal injury, tumor debulking is possible and can be repeated every 3 to 4 days at the endoscopist's discretion.[36] Although earlier reports showed improvement in restoring luminal patency (97%) and oral intake (70%),[37] later comparisons to esophageal stents in an RCT of 65 patients reported disappointing dysphagia scores, higher associated costs and complications (14.7% perforation and/or tracheo-esophageal fistula), as well as a 20.5% need for reintervention due to recurrent dysphagia.[38] Subsequently, with the improvement of endoscopic stents and expansion of available modalities, laser therapy is rarely used in clinical practice.[39] The most recent American Gastroenterological Association (AGA) clinical practice update recommended against the use of laser for esophageal cancer ablation due to the lack of supportive evidence and the availability of better alternatives.[40] The European Society of Gastrointestinal Endoscopy has similar recommendations.[41]

Photodynamic Therapy

Photodynamic therapy (PDT) effects ablation by leveraging a photochemical reaction. A photosensitizing agent (eg, Porfimer sodium) is injected intravenously 40 to 50 hours before endoscopic treatment. The agent accumulates in the tumor at a relatively greater concentration than in normal tissue. Endoscopic application of red light (wavelength of 630 nm) via a noncontact probe to treat the entire tumor activates the agent. A photochemical effect ensues and results in tumor necrosis. Patients undergo repeat endoscopy 2 to 3 days afterward for debridement of necrosed tissue and possible retreatment.[42]

Compared with laser therapy in a prospective trial (118 patients in each group), tumor response persisted for 1 month in 32% of patients with advanced esophageal cancer with equal efficacy for palliation of dysphagia. The rate of adverse events was 92%, and included sunburn, nausea, fever, and pleural effusion.[42] In a retrospective review of 215 patients who underwent palliative PDT for inoperable esophageal cancer, 85% of patients had an improvement in dysphagia, with a reduction dysphagia score (from 3 to 2).[43] In a retrospective study comparing PDT before or after chemoradiation (in case of local recurrence) of esophageal cancer, PDT after chemoradiation was associated with higher rate complications (46.7% vs 8%) including perforations and strictures.[44] Another RCT compared argon plasma coagulation (APC) combined with brachytherapy versus APC with PDT and found that APC with brachytherapy resulted in fewer complications and better QOL than APC with PDT.[45] Patients who undergo PDT are recommended to avoid sunlight for 4 to 6 weeks following the injection of the photosensitizing agent. Therefore, due to the logistical requirements, cost, rates of adverse events, and the lack of compelling treatment advantage, PDT is not commonly used in clinical practice. The most recent AGA clinical practice updates recommended against the use of PDT for esophageal cancer ablation because of lack of supportive evidence and better alternatives.[40] The European Society of Gastrointestinal Endoscopy (ESGE) has similar recommendations.[41]

Argon Plasma Coagulation

APC delivers contact-free electrocoagulation through ionized argon gas. APC was introduced in flexible endoscopy in 1991 and consists of a flexible Teflon tube with a tungsten electrode in a ceramic nozzle at the distal end. The ionized gas is conductive of electricity and allows energy generated by the electrode to be transmitted to the tissue without contact. The electrothermal effect results in superficial tissue necrosis.[46] The necrotic tissue desiccates and is less conductive of electrical energy, thus limiting the effect of APC to the superficial layers. This limits the ablative efficacy of APC per treatment session and contributes to a lower risk of perforation and fistulization.[47] The rate of gas flow varies but is often reported at 2 L/min[48] as studied in a retrospective cohort of 83 patients who underwent palliative endoscopic ablation for inoperable esophageal cancer. Eighty-four percent of patients were ultimately able to eat food normally, with 58% achieving that target after 1 treatment, whereas 26% needing more than 1 treatment. After recanalization of the esophagus, patients underwent retreatment every 3 to 4 weeks.[48] A prospective nonrandomized study compared forced to pulsed APC and found that forced APC worked faster to achieve lumen restoration.[47] APC continues to be an intriguing option for endoscopic palliation in patients with inoperable esophageal cancer because of its simplicity and low risk of adverse event but more studies are needed to elucidate how it can best be used in a manner that offers significant and durable palliation.

Cryoablation

Pressurized liquid nitrogen spray catheter was developed and demonstrated to have both safety and efficacy in the animal model.[49] The ablative effect of cryotherapy mainly relies on the rate of freezing and warming in relation to the kinetics of water through a permeable membrane.[50] The ablative effect stems from direct/immediate cellular injury and delayed vascular injury.[51] At freezing temperatures, extracellular water freezes first and crystallizes. This creates a hyperosmotic extracellular environment and draws out intracellular water, leaving cells dehydrated with an increased electrolyte concentration. With rewarming/thawing, extracellular ice crystals fuse into larger crystals. This causes additional cell damaged by disrupting cell membranes. On further warming, the ice crystals melt and result in a hypotonic extracellular environment. Extracellular water shifts into the damaged cells, which increases cell volumes and may lead to membrane rupture.[52]

With the initial freeze cycle, vasoconstriction occurs with eventual cessation of blood flow. As the treated area thaws, compensatory vasodilation with return of circulation to the now-damaged endothelial cells results in edema, platelet aggregation, cytokine release and microthrombus formation. This results in progressive circulatory failure after thawing, with small vessels and larger arterioles thrombosing within 3 to 4 and 24 hours, respectively. Tissue necrosis follows, largely spares the periphery of frozen tissue volume.[53–55] The low-pressure (<5 psi), noncontact spray allows for freezing mucosal tissue to $-196°$ C. Because of the noncontact delivery method, ablation of topographically variable lesions (ie, flat, nodular and protruding masses) is possible. Although liquid nitrogen is delivered at low pressures, it rapidly expands on transferring to gas at an effective rate of 6 to 7 L/min in a 20-s treatment cycle. Therefore, in addition to the 7-Fr spray catheter, a 20-Fr dual-channel decompression tube with active and passive suction is necessary to be inserted into the lumen throughout the procedure.[56] In application, the decompression tube provides active suction and the spray catheter is extended 0.5 cm to 1 cm from the target lesion. With continuous spray application, a freezing cycle starts when the target lesion becomes frost-white and lasts 20 to 30 seconds. The area is allowed to thaw completely and typically for 45 to 60 seconds.[57] Therefore, a freeze–thaw cycle ranges from 65 to 90 seconds and can be repeated 2 to 3 times depending on indication and endoscopist preference (Video 1).

Cryotherapy is used for palliation in esophageal cancer in different contexts. In patients with localized cancer, cryotherapy is used in an attempt to eradicate local disease and to treat and prevent dysphagia.[58] This primarily is for patients who are not candidates for, or do not want, other local treatments such as radiation. Another context is following chemoradiation—whether in cases of residual cancer in patients who are not surgical candidates, or in cases of disease recurrence after prior complete clinical response. Data from early adopters suggest that more superficial cancers have a higher chance of eradication with cryotherapy. In a study of patients with esophageal cancer (ranging from T1 to T4) and underwent cryotherapy, subsets of the above cohorts were retrospectively reviewed among 10 medical centers.[59] Seventy-nine patients with esophageal cancer who were ineligible for, had ineffective, and/or refused other treatments underwent cryotherapy with the express goal of tumor palliation. Treatment protocols were consistent with earlier reports with freezing cycle of

20 seconds, followed by at least 45 seconds of thawing, for 3 times. Treatment was repeated every 4 to 6 weeks until local tumor eradication as determined endoscopically. Esophageal biopsies were performed every 3 to 6 months after completion of ablation. Safety analysis of a total of 332 treatments in the 79 patients had no serious adverse events such as perforation or hemorrhage. Ten patients (13%) had benign strictures, 9 of whom were noted to have had narrowing of the esophageal lumen before cryotherapy. Twenty (27%) patients had posttreatment pain and required the use of narcotics. Efficacy was only assessed in 49 patients because the remaining 30 patients were still receiving cryotherapy. Thirty (61.2%) of 49 patients had a complete response of luminal disease with cryotherapy when followed for a mean of 10.6 months. Most of the patients had T1 tumors (36 out of 49—73.5%). Endoscopic remission was achieved in 72.2% of all T1 tumors, and in 18 out of 24 (75%) of T1a tumors. Eight patients underwent concurrent treatments, which included endoscopic resection and/or ablation with APC. The authors examined the rates of complete response when excluding the 8 patients with concurrent treatments and found that 27 out of 41 (66%) had complete response of luminal disease. Sixteen subjects had T2 disease, and only 3 subjects attained a complete response. Two patients had T3 disease, and both received chemotherapy and radiotherapy before cryotherapy. One of the patients required 8 treatments before biopsies demonstrating luminal absence of cancer. Therefore, this cohort recapitulated the promising potential of an adjunct and/or salvage modality, without concern for serious adverse effects.[57] Based on clinical observation and emerging data, it is our opinion that cryotherapy may be more effective with an intensive dosing schedule. A phase 1 dose–frequency escalation of up to 3 sessions of liquid nitrogen spray cryotherapy during the neoadjuvant chemoradiation setting for 14 patients with locally advanced esophageal cancer had no grade 2 or 3 toxicity, and had mean dysphagia score improvement of 0.4, 0.7, and 0.6 at 1 week following the first, second, and third sessions.[60]

Cryotherapy is also useful in the palliation of patients with inoperable disease. A multicenter retrospective study specifically assessed dysphagia palliation in stage III and IV esophageal cancer.[61] A total of 49 patients (83.7% stage IV) underwent a total of 120 treatments (mean of 2.4 per patient). Each tumor site was frozen for 20 to 30 seconds for 2 to 3 cycles per site, allowing a minimum of 45 seconds for thawing. Retreatment occurred every 2 to 12 weeks depending on the severity of dysphagia and the clinical response to treatment. Dysphagia was assessed on the 5-point scale (see **Box 1**). Before cryotherapy, only 8.2% had dysphagia scores of less than 1. After the last cryotherapy, 40.8% had dysphagia scores less than 1. Of the 49 patients, the mean dysphagia score improved from 2.6 to 1.7 ($P < .001$). Some important observations also included a higher likelihood of improved dysphagia score in patients aged younger than 60 years and those without prior local treatment. The total time of freeze per site and the number of cycles were not associated with a change in dysphagia scores. Comparable to earlier reports, there were minor adverse events, which included chest pain, stricture formation requiring dilations, and transient bradycardia. Another patient developed perforation related to dilation before cryotherapy, which was not performed in favor of a fully covered stent. This account demonstrated the potential of cryotherapy in palliating esophageal cancer that is locally advanced and/or metastatic.

A more recent prospective, multicenter cohort study evaluated 55 patients who had inoperable esophageal cancer with plans to receive systemic treatment.[7] A mean 3.3 cryotherapy sessions per patient was associated with an improvement in mean dysphagia score from 1.9 to 1.2 ($P = .005$), as well as EORTC QOL improvement from 35 to 29 ($P < .001$). Patients who received intensive cryotherapy (defined as 2 or more cryotherapy sessions within 3 weeks) were more likely to have a bigger dysphagia score improvement (1.2 vs 0.2 points difference; $P < .005$). There was a trend toward improved dysphagia with concurrent (defined as within 48 hours) cryotherapy and systemic chemotherapy. The rate of procedure-related adverse events that were grade 3 (CTCAE) or higher was 1%, and included hospitalization for postprocedural abdominal pain and abdominal distension. In the same study, a few patients received multiple sessions (eg, 4 cryotherapy sessions within 5 weeks) and were free of dysphagia. Some patients with intensive therapy show improvement in luminal disease despite progression of disease elsewhere (**Fig. 1**). The rationale for intensive therapy is based on animal data demonstrating that cryotherapy combined with systemic therapy decreases cancer volume up until the 4-week mark, when cancer volume begins to increase again.[62] Therefore, treating patients at shorter intervals is likely to have a cumulative effect of decreasing cancer volume. Similarly, animal data suggest that combining cryotherapy treatment within 48 hours of systemic therapy is likely to result in a higher response rate than in a longer window.[63] It is our practice to treat patients with inoperable esophageal cancer with 3 sessions of cryotherapy 3 weeks apart, typically within 2 days before a dose of systemic therapy, and then reevaluate their response.

In the recent prospective study, dysphagia and QOL improved with cryotherapy, with most patients being able to lie flat without reflux symptoms. Of the 55 patients, 13 required another intervention for dysphagia and only 2 required stenting.[7] Although this study did not compare cryotherapy to esophageal stents, the latter is known to cause significant reflux when placed across the gastroesophageal junction.[64] A retrospective review of 56 patients who underwent cryotherapy for palliation of dysphagia related to esophageal cancer found that more than 75% of the cohort did not require subsequent palliative stenting (mean follow-up of over 2 years).[65] This suggests that in cases where cryotherapy is feasible, esophageal stenting may not be needed.

Finally, there are emerging data on cryotherapy for dysphagia palliation in the neoadjuvant setting. A 2-center study on the neoadjuvant effects of cryotherapy at the time of endoscopic diagnosis evaluated dysphagia score improvement and clinical complete response rate after chemoradiation.[66] Dysphagia was assessed on a 5-point scale (see **Box 1**). A total of 21 patients with dysphagia underwent initial endoscopies for diagnosis and received 2 cycles of 20-second freeze per site, with 60-second thaw cycles. A median of 2 sites were treated. Median dysphagia score improved by 1 at 1 week and 0.5 at 2 weeks. Chemoradiation was initiated at a median of 27 days after cryotherapy. A local complete response was observed in 67% of those patients, whereas 56% of patients had complete clinical response with no evidence of tumor on repeat biopsies or PET scan. These findings raised the possibility of synergy between cryotherapy and chemoradiation.

Esophageal Stenting

Esophageal prostheses to maintain luminal patency have been examined since the 1840s. In 1959, Celestine introduced plastic stents that are placed through a laparotomy with an open gastrostomy for palliation of esophageal cancer.[67] In 1977, a technique for introducing the stent endoscopically was introduced and was popularized because it avoided laparotomy and complications thereof.[68] In the early 1980s, self-expanding metal stents (SEMS) began to be used for palliation of malignant esophageal stenoses.[69] The 2 major types of SEMS are made from a nickel-titanium alloy (nitinol) or stainless steel. These inert materials are erosion resistant and nonallergenic. The nitinol stents are stored inside a sheath in a constricted form and have thermal shape memory that expands at body temperature allowing them to reexpand when

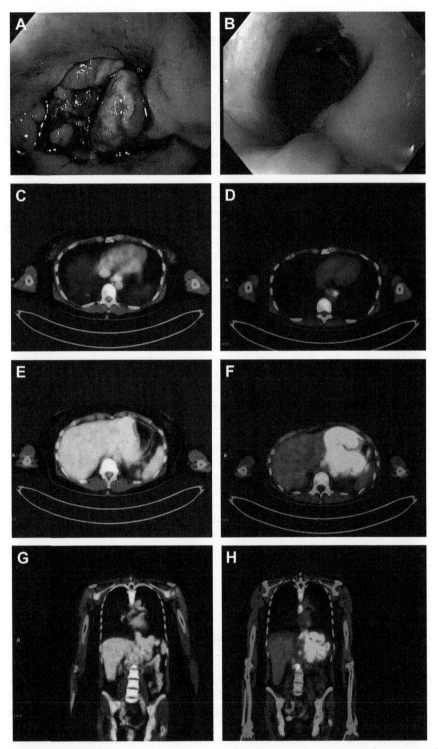

Fig. 1. The left side shows endoscopic images and positron emission tomography–computed tomography (PET CT) cuts before cryotherapy and chemotherapy, whereas the right side depicts corresponding representation after cryotherapy and chemotherapy. (*A*) Endoscopic

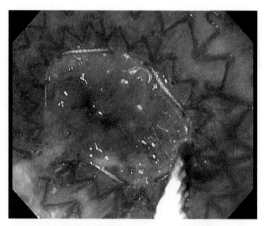

Fig. 2. Endoscopic appearance following esophageal stent placement.

deployed across an area obstructed by tumor. Most stents used today are either fully covered (FCSEMS) (**Figs. 2** and **3**) or partially covered stents (PCSEMS).[39] FCSEMS have a membrane that spans the entire stent and thus prevents tissue ingrowth (whether malignant or reactive). Various polymer-coated materials were developed to mitigate tissue ingrowth; however, stent migration became a common complication occurring up to 36.3%.[70] PCSEMS have part of the stent uncovered, often with a flared tip allowing tissue to grow through the interstices to help anchor the stent with the aim of decreasing stent migration. However, no differences have been found in dysphagia or rates of migration.[71] Different FCSEMS fixation techniques could mitigate the risk of migration. For example, endoscopic suturing of FCSEMS was found to reduce clinically significant stent migration rates (9.4% vs 39.4%).[72,73] Similarly, through-the-scope and over-the-scope[74,75] clips have been reported to have stent migration rates as low as 3.2%. In addition to technical feasibility and success, palliative stenting can significantly improve dysphagia and functional QOL.[76] Conversely, some studies have shown worsening of QOL with stents compared with other modalities, despite improvement in dysphagia.[22,38,77]

Stents have been shown to promptly improve dysphagia by up to 3 points, and this modality often allows patients with severe obstruction to resume oral intake within hours from the procedure.[71] However, stents have a high rate of adverse events. The most common serious adverse events include migration, pain, and recurrent obstruction from tumor/tissue ingrowth or overgrowth. Other less common but potentially serious adverse events include bleeding, perforation, and fistula formation.[78] The most common adverse event following stent placement is chest pain.[79] If a stent

appearance of the distal esophageal tumor before cryo and chemotherapy, (*B*) Endoscopic appearance of the distal esophageal tumor after cryo and chemotherapy, (*C*) distal esophagus activity before cryo and chemotherapy on PET-CT, (*D*) distal esophagus activity after cryo and chemotherapy on PET-CT, (*E*) gastric body activity before cryo and chemotherapy on cross sectional imaging on PET-CT, (*F*) gastric body activity after cryo and chemotherapy on cross sectional imaging on PET-CT, (*G*) gastric body activity before cryo and chemotherapy on coronal imaging on PET-CT, (*H*) gastric body activity after cryo and chemotherapy on coronal imaging on PET-CT.

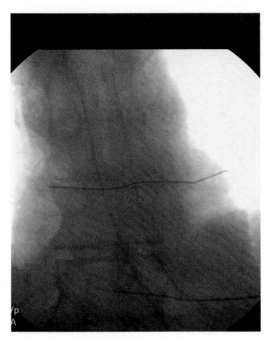

Fig. 3. Fluoroscopic appearance of esophageal stent placed.

traverses the gastroesophageal junction, acid reflux occurs. It is recommended that patients elevate the head of the bed and take proton pump inhibitors (PPIs) twice daily. Antireflux esophageal stents with a 1-way valve design have not had a definitive advantage in preventing reflux symptoms when compared with "open" stents combined with PPIs.[80]

Overall, the technical success rate of stents is more than 90% and approaches 100% with experienced endoscopists. Improvement in dysphagia is prompt and can be up to 3 points on a 5-point scale. The influence on QOL seems positive, although some data show mixed results. The risks of adverse events due to stent placements are as follows: migration (5%–30%), stent obstruction by tumor (5%–30%), stent obstruction by food (2%–10%), chest pain (2%–20%), and bleeding (3%–10%). The data do not favor a particular stent type (eg, FCSEMS vs PCSEMS). The NCCN recommends removal if an esophageal stent results in severe uncontrolled pain. Therefore, we favor using FCSEMS over PCSEMS because the former is easier to remove if needed.

Combination Therapies of Different Modalities

In current clinical practice, many patients receive multiple modalities for cancer palliation either simultaneously or sequentially. It is therefore important to understand how different modalities may interact to affect palliation. Patients with inoperable cancer can be locally advanced or metastatic. In patients with locally advanced disease and are not surgical candidates, systemic therapy is often combined with radiation given that the chance of complete clinical response was 29% in the CROSS trial.[33] Patients with metastatic disease have shorter survival than patients with locally advanced disease. Because there is no chance of complete clinical response, palliation is the focus of therapy. Systemic therapy is the standard of care for patients with inoperable esophageal cancer given its improved survival. It is offered to patients who have a good functional status to tolerate it. As discussed earlier, longer term palliation of dysphagia requires more than systemic therapy—often multiple modalities. Cryotherapy seems to be one of the safest options in patients with mild-to-moderate symptoms. EBRT with chemotherapy versus EBRT alone did not show palliation benefit. Therefore, when used, EBRT is used, it is performed when patients hold chemotherapy or undergo a chemotherapy break. Brachytherapy with chemotherapy has also been associated with an increased risk of adverse events, especially fistula formation.

There is no clear consensus on the utility of EBRT in combination with stents. In a multicenter RCT, patients who underwent stent placement were randomized to typical stent care versus the addition of EBRT (20 Gy in 5 fractions or 30 Gy in 10 fractions) after stent placement.[81] The addition of radiotherapy did not reduce dysphagia deterioration per the EORTC, which occurred in 49% and 45%, respectively. Overall survival was comparable at 19.7 versus 18.9 weeks for the added radiotherapy versus stent only. The mean time for a bleeding event was longer for the added radiotherapy group than for the stent-only group 65.9 weeks versus 49 weeks, respectively, with an adjusted subhazard ratio of 0.52 [95% CI 0.28–0.97, $P = .038$]. There were no differences in the rate of stent complications or time to, or need for, reinterventions between groups. Therefore, other than for a subset of patients who may be clinically considered to be at an increased risk for bleeding, the addition of radiotherapy after stent placement did not seem to achieve additional palliative benefit.[81] Radioactive stents, however, seem to be associated with longer survival and stent patency.[82] However, these are not widely available. More studies are needed before they are widely adopted.

A prospective randomized trial evaluated brachytherapy (8 Gy × 3) alone versus brachytherapy preceded by SEMS placement in a total of 41 patients with inoperable esophageal cancer. In the combination group, dysphagia improved with a mean score change of 1, compared with a mean score change of 0 in the brachytherapy-only group.[83]

Palliation in the Neoadjuvant Setting

Patients who are receiving neoadjuvant treatment with potential for surgery can have significant dysphagia requiring some intervention. In these patients, it is imperative to have a multidisciplinary discussion before offering them endoscopic palliative options. For example, for nutrition support, stents are often avoided. In such cases, jejunal feeding tubes are preferred to avoid the potential limitation of gastric tubes impeding the ability to use the stomach as a conduit following esophagectomy.[8] Although there are no clear data on this topic, the NCCN guidelines also recommend against stenting in such patients because adverse events may influence the ability of undergoing surgery. It is highly advisable that multidisciplinary planning precedes any intervention in such cases. Cryotherapy is being studied in this paradigm and could prove to be a viable option to improve the oncological outcome as well as palliate dysphagia. Pilot studies are forthcoming, and more studies are necessary to guide this potential.

In conclusion, esophageal cancer palliation is complex and should be done in a multidisciplinary team. It continues to be dependent on local familiarity and available expertise. Systemic therapy is the standard of care, and often needs to be augmented by another form of therapy. Stenting has a prompt influence on dysphagia with possible positive influence on QOL. It is preferred in severe dysphagia and in patients with an expected short-term survival. It is less preferred in patients with an expected longer-term survival, as adverse events can be as high as 50%. Brachytherapy is an option in patients who have a longer expected survival but it is not widely available. Laser and PDT have fallen out of favor due to the rate of adverse events and the lack of superiority over other available options. Cryotherapy is a relatively newer modality that is showing promise and seems to have one of the lowest adverse event rates. Emerging data can help guide how cryotherapy can optimize outcomes. We favor it in patients with mild-to-moderate symptoms. Palliation in the neoadjuvant setting should be offered only as a part of a multidisciplinary discussion of risks and benefits. This is important as adverse events from an intervention can influence oncological outcomes and render a potentially resectable patient unresectable.

SUMMARY

The management of inoperable esophageal cancer is complex. The objective of progression-free survival needs to be balanced with palliation and global HRQOL. Dysphagia scoring has been commonly used but the implication on HRQOL can be difficult to ascertain given the differences in metrics evaluated among different studies. Because more studies adopt validated metrics for disease-specific outcomes, for example, the EORTC, more meaningful comparisons can inform providers and patients on individualizing treatment. In our experience, we favor esophageal stents for palliation of severe dysphagia with obstruction. For mild-to-moderate dysphagia, we favor cryotherapy. Given our clinical experience and emerging evidence, we counsel patients on leveraging the combination of chemotherapy ideally within 48 hours from cryotherapy to maximize tumor response. We favor cryotherapy over APC to maximize the submucosal depth of tissue ablation, given the invasive nature of inoperable esophageal cancer. Ultimately, as endoscopists develop expertise at the technical level, the combination of systemic and/or RT through multidisciplinary collaboration will afford patients with different protocols that may be individualized according to objectives.

CLINICS CARE POINTS

- Esophageal cancer palliation is complex and should be done in a multidisciplinary team.
- Available modalities depend on local and available expertise.
- Systemic therapy is the standard of care and can be augmented by other modalities.
- Esophageal stenting has a prompt impact on dysphagia with possible positive influence on QOL.
- We favor esophageal stenting in severe dysphagia and in patients with short-term expected survival.
- In patients with longer term expected survival, brachytherapy is a durable option. It is limited by complex logistics and not being widely available.
- Cryotherapy is a new modality that is promising with one of the lowest adverse event rates.
- Emerging data on cryotherapy can help further optimize outcomes.
- We favor cryotherapy in patients with mild-to-moderate symptoms of dysphagia.
- Palliation in neoadjuvant setting should be very carefully planned within a multidisciplinary team because adverse events from intervention could render a potentially resectable patient unresectable.

DISCLOSURE

Y.Y. Soliman: no relevant disclosures. M. Kundranda: Research funding (to institution): Bayer, BMS, and chronix. Consulting: AstraZeneca, BMS, United States, Steris, Bayer, Germany, and Exact Sciences. T. Kachaamy: Steris, Pentax, Microtech, Medtronic, Boston Scientific, International private bank-intellectual property partnership.

SUPPLEMENTARY DATA

Supplementary data related to this article can be found online at https://doi.org/10.1016/j.giec.2023.07.003.

REFERENCES

1. Uhlenhopp DJ, Then EO, Sunkara T, et al. Epidemiology of esophageal cancer: update in global trends, etiology and risk factors. Clin J Gastroenterol 2020; 13(6):1010–21.
2. Siegel RL, Miller KD, Wagle NS, et al. Cancer statistics, 2023. CA Cancer J Clin 2023;73(1):17–48.
3. Siegel RL, Miller KD, Fuchs HE, et al. Cancer statistics, 2022. CA. A Cancer Journal for Clinicians 2022;72(1):7–33.
4. CROSS Study Group, Eyck BM, van Lanschot JJB, et al. Ten-Year Outcome of Neoadjuvant Chemoradiotherapy Plus Surgery for Esophageal Cancer: The Randomized Controlled CROSS Trial. J Clin Oncol : official journal of the American Society of Clinical Oncology 2021;39(18):1995–2004.
5. Reynolds JV, Preston SR, O'Neill B, et al. Neo-AEGIS (Neoadjuvant trial in Adenocarcinoma of the Esophagus and Esophago-Gastric Junction International Study): Preliminary results of phase III RCT of CROSS versus perioperative chemotherapy (Modified MAGIC or FLOT protocol). (NCT01726452). J Clin Orthod 2021;39(15_suppl):4004.
6. Depypere L, Thomas M, Moons J, et al. Analysis of patients scheduled for neoadjuvant therapy followed by surgery for esophageal cancer, who never made it to esophagectomy. World J Surg Oncol 2019;17:89.
7. Kachaamy T, Sharma NR, Shah T, et al. A Prospective Multicenter Study to Evaluate the Impact of Cryotherapy on Dysphagia and Quality of Life in Patients with Inoperable Esophageal Cancer. Endoscopy 2023. https://doi.org/10.1055/a-2105-2177.
8. Ajani JA, Barthel JS, Bentrem DJ, et al. Esophageal and Esophagogastric Junction Cancers. J Natl Compr Canc Netw 2011;9(8):830–87. Referenced with permission from the NCCN Clinical Practice Guidelines in Oncology (NCCN Guidelines®) for Guideline Name V.2.2023. © National Comprehensive Cancer Network, Inc. 2023. All rights reserved. Accessed June 30, 2023. To view the most recent and complete version of the guideline, go online to NCCN.org.
9. Mellow MH, Pinkas H. Endoscopic therapy for esophageal carcinoma with Nd:YAG laser: prospective evaluation of efficacy, complications, and survival. Gastrointest Endosc 1984;30(6):334–9.
10. Blazeby JM, Conroy T, Hammerlid E, et al. Clinical and psychometric validation of an EORTC questionnaire module, the EORTC QLQ-OES18, to assess quality of life in patients with oesophageal cancer. Eur J Cancer 2003; 39(10):1384–94.

patients with malignant dysphagia (CONSORT 1a) (Revised II). Am J Gastroenterol 2011;106(9):1612–20.

46. Wahab PJ, Mulder CJ, den Hartog G, et al. Argon plasma coagulation in flexible gastrointestinal endoscopy: pilot experiences. Endoscopy 1997;29(3):176–81.

47. Eickhoff A, Jakobs R, Schilling D, et al. Prospective nonrandomized comparison of two modes of argon beamer (APC) tumor desobstruction: effectiveness of the new pulsed APC versus forced APC. Endoscopy 2007;39(7):637–42.

48. Heindorff H, Wøjdemann M, Bisgaard T, et al. Endoscopic palliation of inoperable cancer of the oesophagus or cardia by argon electrocoagulation. Scand J Gastroenterol 1998;33(1):21–3.

49. Johnston CM, Schoenfeld LP, Mysore JV, et al. Endoscopic spray cryotherapy: a new technique for mucosal ablation in the esophagus. Gastrointest Endosc 1999; 50(1):86–92.

50. Mazur P. Kinetics of Water Loss from Cells at Subzero Temperatures and the Likelihood of Intracellular Freezing. J Gen Physiol 1963;47(2):347–69.

51. Theodorescu D. Cancer Cryotherapy: Evolution and Biology. Rev Urol 2004; 6(Suppl 4):S9–19.

52. Gage AA, Baust J. Mechanisms of Tissue Injury in Cryosurgery. Cryobiology 1998;37(3):171–86.

53. Adams-Ray J, Bellman S. Vascular reactions after experimental cold injury; a microangiographic study of rabbit ears. Angiology 1956;7(4):339–67.

54. Bowers WD, Hubbard RW, Daum RC, et al. Ultrastructural studies of muscle cells and vascular endothelium immediately after freeze-thaw injury. Cryobiology 1973; 10(1):9–21.

55. Giampapa VC, Oh C, Aufses AH. The vascular effect of cold injury. Cryobiology 1981;18(1):49–54.

56. Dumot JA, Greenwald BD. Cryotherapy for Barrett's esophagus: does the gas really matter? Endoscopy. Published online March 2011;29:432–3.

57. Greenwald BD, Dumot JA, Horwhat JD, et al. Safety, tolerability, and efficacy of endoscopic low-pressure liquid nitrogen spray cryotherapy in the esophagus. Dis Esophagus 2010;23(1):13–9.

58. Spiritos Z, Mekaroonkamol P, El-Rayes BF, et al. Long-Term Survival in Stage IV Esophageal Adenocarcinoma with Chemoradiation and Serial Endoscopic Cryoablation. Clin Endosc 2017;50(5):491–4.

59. Greenwald BD, Dumot JA, Abrams JA, et al. Endoscopic spray cryotherapy for esophageal cancer: safety and efficacy. Gastrointest Endosc 2010;71(4):686–93.

60. Shah T, Spataro J, Mutha P, et al. PHASE 1 DOSE-FREQUENCY ESCALATION STUDY OF NEOADJUVANT CRYOTHERAPY IN LOCALLY ADVANCED ESOPHAGEAL CANCER. Gastrointest Endosc 2023;97(6):AB1106–7.

61. Kachaamy T, Prakash R, Kundranda M, et al. Liquid nitrogen spray cryotherapy for dysphagia palliation in patients with inoperable esophageal cancer. Gastrointest Endosc 2018;88(3):447–55.

62. Forest V, Peoc'h M, Campos L, et al. Benefit of a combined treatment of cryotherapy and chemotherapy on tumour growth and late cryo-induced angiogenesis in a non-small-cell lung cancer model. Lung Cancer 2006;54(1): 79–86.

63. Forest V, Hadjeres R, Bertrand R, et al. Optimisation and molecular signalling of apoptosis in sequential cryotherapy and chemotherapy combination in human A549 lung cancer xenografts in SCID mice. Br J Cancer 2009;100(12): 1896–902.

64. Sabharwal T, Gulati MS, Fotiadis N, et al. Randomised comparison of the FerX Ella antireflux stent and the ultraflex stent: proton pump inhibitor combination for prevention of post-stent reflux in patients with esophageal carcinoma involving the esophago-gastric junction. J Gastroenterol Hepatol 2008;23(5):723–8.

65. Hanada Y, Leggett CL, Iyer PG, et al. Spray cryotherapy prevents need for palliative stenting in patients with esophageal cancer-associated dysphagia. Dis Esophagus 2022;35(1):doab051.

66. Shah T, Kushnir V, Mutha P, et al. Neoadjuvant cryotherapy improves dysphagia and may impact remission rates in advanced esophageal cancer. Endosc Int Open 2019;7(11):E1522–7.

67. Celestin LR. Permanent Intubation in Inoperable Cancer of the Oesophagus and Cardia. Ann R Coll Surg Engl 1959;25(2):165–70.

68. Atkinson M, Ferguson R. Fibreoptic endoscopic palliative intubation of inoperable oesophagogastric neoplasms. Br Med J 1977;1(6056):266–7.

69. Frimberger E. Expanding spiral–a new type of prosthesis for the palliative treatment of malignant esophageal stenoses. Endoscopy 1983;15(Suppl 1): 213–4.

70. So H, Ahn JY, Han S, et al. Efficacy and Safety of Fully Covered Self-Expanding Metal Stents for Malignant Esophageal Obstruction. Dig Dis Sci 2018;63(1): 234–41.

71. Wang C, Wei H, Li Y. Comparison of fully-covered vs partially covered self-expanding metallic stents for palliative treatment of inoperable esophageal malignancy: a systematic review and meta-analysis. BMC Cancer 2020;20:73.

72. Bick BL, Imperiale TF, Johnson CS, et al. Endoscopic suturing of esophageal fully covered self-expanding metal stents reduces rates of stent migration. Gastrointest Endosc 2017;86(6):1015–21.

73. Vanbiervliet G, Filippi J, Karimdjee BS, et al. The role of clips in preventing migration of fully covered metallic esophageal stents: a pilot comparative study. Surg Endosc 2012;26(1):53–9.

74. Watanabe K, Hikichi T, Nakamura J, et al. Feasibility of esophageal stent fixation with an over-the-scope-clip for malignant esophageal strictures to prevent migration. Endosc Int Open 2017;5(11):E1044–9.

75. Manta R, Del Nero L, Todd B, et al. Newly designed OTS Clip for preventing fully-covered self-expandable metal stent migration in the gastrointestinal tract. Endosc Int Open 2023;11(3):E284–7.

76. Madhusudhan C, Saluja SS, Pal S, et al. Palliative stenting for relief of dysphagia in patients with inoperable esophageal cancer: impact on quality of life. Dis Esophagus 2009;22(4):331–6.

77. Shenfine J, McNamee P, Steen N, et al. A pragmatic randomised controlled trial of the cost-effectiveness of palliative therapies for patients with inoperable oesophageal cancer. Health Technol Assess 2005;9(5):1–121, iii.

78. Kang Y. A Review of Self-Expanding Esophageal Stents for the Palliation Therapy of Inoperable Esophageal Malignancies. BioMed Res Int 2019;2019:9265017.

79. Diamantis G, Scarpa M, Bocus P, et al. Quality of life in patients with esophageal stenting for the palliation of malignant dysphagia. World J Gastroenterol 2011; 17(2):144–50.

80. Sasso JGRJ, de Moura DTH, Proença IM, et al. Anti-reflux versus conventional self-expanding metal stents in the palliation of esophageal cancer: A systematic review and meta-analysis. Endosc Int Open 2022;10(10):E1406–16.

81. Adamson D, Byrne A, Porter C, et al. Palliative radiotherapy after oesophageal cancer stenting (ROCS): a multicentre, open-label, phase 3 randomised controlled trial. Lancet Gastroenterol Hepatol 2021;6(4):292–303.
82. Yang ZM, Geng HT, Wu H. Radioactive Stent for Malignant Esophageal Obstruction: A Meta-Analysis of Randomized Controlled Trials. J Laparoendosc Adv Surg Tech 2021;31(7):783–9.
83. Amdal CD, Jacobsen AB, Sandstad B, et al. Palliative brachytherapy with or without primary stent placement in patients with oesophageal cancer, a randomised phase III trial. Radiother Oncol 2013;107(3):428–33.

Endoscopic Treatment of Gastric Outlet Obstruction

Andrew Canakis, DO[a], Shayan S. Irani, MD[b],*

KEYWORDS

- EUS-guided gastroenterostomy • Lumen-apposing metal stent
- Endoscopic balloon dilation • Enteral stenting • Surgical gastrojejunostomy
- Benign GOO • Malignant GOO

KEY POINTS

- Management of gastric outlet obstruction (GOO) depends on if benign or malignant etiology, underlying anatomy, surgical candidacy, and available expertise and should be done in a multidisciplinary approach.
- Endoluminal stenting with a self-expandable metal stent is an effective modality to treat malignant GOO in patients with a life expectancy less than 3 months.
- Compared with surgery, EUS-GE is associated with shorter times to oral intake, shorter postintervention length of stay, and maybe fewer adverse events.
- Refractory cases of benign GOO may be managed by EUS-GE in nonoperative candidates.

INTRODUCTION

Gastric outlet obstruction (GOO) is the clinical manifestation of a mechanical obstruction at the antro-pyloric region or proximal small bowel. It can result from benign or malignant causes, and patients often present with early satiety, worsening heartburn, epigastric pain, nausea, vomiting, and/or weight loss. Symptom onset and progression varies based on the degree of mechanical blockage, where extensive obstruction can quickly lead to limited per os (PO) intake, volume depletion, and malnutrition. In cases of malignant GOO, such a sequela may disrupt chemotherapy treatment options and affect one's quality of life. Consequently, managing this obstruction is paramount in order to reduce symptoms and reestablish PO intake. In this review, we will discuss the evolution, current perspective, and future considerations of endoscopic approaches for relieving GOO.

[a] Division of Gastroenterology & Hepatology, University of Maryland Medical Center, 22 South Greene Street, Baltimore, MD 21201, USA; [b] Division of Gastroenterology and Hepatology, Virginia Mason Medical Center, 1100 Ninth Avenue, Mailstop: C3-GAS, Seattle, WA 98101, USA
* Corresponding author.
E-mail address: shayan.irani@virginiamason.org

Gastrointest Endoscopy Clin N Am 34 (2024) 111–125
https://doi.org/10.1016/j.giec.2023.08.005
1052-5157/24/© 2023 Elsevier Inc. All rights reserved.

Cause and Epidemiology

The exact incidence of benign and malignant causes of GOO is unknown. Historically, peptic ulcer disease was the leading cause of GOO; however, with an increased use of acid suppression therapy and recognition/treatment of *Helicobacter pylori* infection, its incidence has significantly declined down to 5%.[1] Other benign causes may be related to caustic ingestion, nonsteroidal anti-inflammatory drugs use, Crohn's disease, post-surgical scarring/adhesion, chronic pancreatitis, superior mesenteric artery syndrome, or even retroperitoneal fibrosis.[2] Malignancy is now the leading cause of GOO accounting for 50% to 80% of cases, primarily from gastric and periampullary cancers.[3] It is estimated that up to 20% of patients with pancreatic cancer develop GOO.[4]

Management

The goal of treatment is to relieve and palliate obstruction so patients can resume PO intake in a timely manner. There are endoscopic and surgical treatment options. Decisions are typically based on the underlying cause, degree of obstruction, patients' performance status, anatomy, and prognosis. Benign intrinsic causes are typically treated with endoscopic dilation, sometimes with temporary covered metal stents (fully covered self-expanding metal stent [FCSEMS] and lumen-apposing metal stent [LAMS]) and more definitely with surgical gastrojejunostomy (SGJ).[5] In the context of malignant GOO, many patients suffer debilitating symptoms that require long-lasting durable palliation. Traditionally, SGJ has provided reliable outcomes and symptomatic relief although its use is associated with a significant morbidity and mortality.[6] In cases of advanced disease, patients may not be operative candidates and a less-invasive alternative is needed. Consequently, enteral stenting (ES) emerged as a means to provide short-term palliation with a technical success of greater than 95% and clinical success of 75% to 85%. However, it is associated with higher rates of reintervention from stent dysfunction (tissue/tumor ingrowth/overgrowth).[7] A multitude of comparative studies between SGJ and ES were done to determine the optimal management strategy.[8–11]

In recent years, the therapeutic application of endoscopic ultrasound-guided gastroenterostomy (EUS-GE) has emerged as a novel minimally invasive alternative to palliate obstruction in patients who may not be ideal operative candidates.[12] Understanding and comparing all 3 approaches is critical because optimizing therapy based on individual patient selection factors can enhance the technical outcomes, improve the clinical response and limit adverse events (**Fig. 1**).

Surgical Gastrojejunostomy

Historically, SGJ was the mainstay of treatment. Conversion from an open to laparoscopic approach improved clinical and operative outcomes. The anastomosis can be anteocolic or retrocolic, with the former being used due to less instances of internal herniation. Although there is no clear survival benefit between an open and laparoscopic SGJ, the laparoscopic method is linked to better outcomes.[13] Compared with open-SGJ, laparoscopic-SGJ has been associated with decreased hospital length of stay (LOS), less intraoperative bleeding, faster time to solid food intake, and less use of postoperative opioids.[6,14,15] Yet this operation is associated with a significant morbidity and some mortality. Postoperative complications from laparoscopic-SGJ include anastomotic leaks, delayed gastric emptying, and postoperative ileus.[16,17] Additionally, hypoalbuminemia can worsen wound and anastomosis healing following SGJ.[14]

Endoluminal Stenting

In an effort to reduce the morbidity of SGJ, endoluminal stenting with a self-expandable metal stent (SEMS) emerged as an effective modality to treat malignant

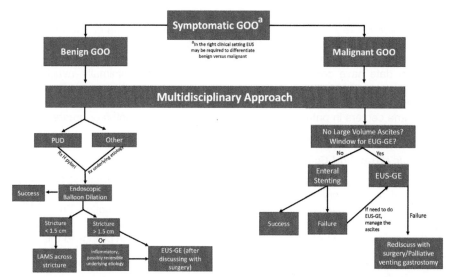

Fig. 1. In the right clinical setting endoscopic ultrasound may be required to differentiate benign versus malignant.

GOO, in patients with a shorter life expectancy or who may not be operative candidates. Under endoscopic and/or fluoroscopic guidance, an over the wire or through the scope technique is used to deploy the stent across the stricture. A therapeutic forward viewing endoscope allows easiest deployment but a duodenoscope can be used as well. Duodenal SEMS are typically uncovered although in some countries partially covered and fully covered versions are available. Studies have found no major differences in technical or clinical outcomes between stent types.[18–20] In general, uncovered stents are preferred in cases of malignant GOO and should not be used in benign indications. Two meta-analyses comparing covered versus uncovered SEMS found that while covered stents were associated with a lower occlusion risk, the higher rates of stent migration offset these benefits.[20,21] Factors associated with stent failure have been examined in multiple studies, in which carcinomatosis with ascites, Eastern Cooperative Oncology Group (ECOG) status of 3 or greater and distal gastro-duodenal stricture with 3 or greater stricture sites were predictors of clinical failure while initiation of chemotherapy after stent therapy was protective.[22–26]

Comparing surgical gastrojejunostomy to endoscopic enteral stenting
Comparisons between SGJ and ES have been well studied. A recent meta-analysis of 31 studies with 2444 patients with malignant GOO (SGJ 1076, 1368 ES) demonstrated no differences in clinical success, although the SGJ group was associated with higher technical success rate and lower reintervention rates.[27] There was no difference in adverse events or clinical success between the 2 groups. Another comparative meta-analysis of 39 studies (SGJ 2116, ES 3128) showed that ES group had a shorter LOS and time to resumption of oral intake while the SGJ patients had long survival (by 25 days) and lower risks of reintervention.[28] In addition to decreased LOS, ES is also associated with lower costs (US$15,366 vs US$27,391).[29] A single center retrospective study, using a propensity score analysis, found that compared with ES (n = 183), SGJ (n = 127) significantly increased the mean patency duration (169.2 vs 96.5 days, $P < .001$) and survival time (193.4 vs 119.9 days, $P<.001$) in patients with malignant

obstruction.[30] However, studies such as this should be interpreted with caution because there is likely selection bias in outcomes where patients not fit for surgery are undergoing ES and being compared with those with better preoperative performance scores, as indicated by the differences in ECOG scores. Furthermore, most studies to date have combined SGJ to include open and minimally invasive approaches, which could further influence results and create more heterogeneity in study outcomes. In general, before the availability of EUS-GJ, SGJ was preferred at many high-volume centers in patients with a life expectancy of 3 months or greater due to its long-term durability and fewer reinterventions.

Endoscopic Ultrasound-Guided Gastroenterostomy

EUS-GE has emerged as novel, minimally invasive technique to treat GOO through deployment of a cautery-enhanced LAMS to create a transmural tract between the stomach and small bowel as a means to bypass the point of obstruction. Endoscopic gastroenterostomy was initially introduced in a preclinical study in 2002, yet it was not until the introduction of LAMS in 2012 when Binmoeller and Shah proposed this novel technique in a porcine animal model that led way to a feasible and safe adaptation in humans.[31,32] The first clinical experience in the United States involved 10 patients (3 malignant, 7 benign) in 2015, where there was a 90% technical success rate with no adverse events—clinical success was achieved in all patients.[33] Since then, EUS-GE has been adopted rapidly with evolving techniques and reliable outcomes. In fact, one group analyzed the learning curve (defined by procedure time) for performing EUS-GE using the freehand technique with cautery-enhanced LAMS during a 5-year period in 73 patients with one experienced operator.[34] Using a cumulative sum analysis they found that proficiency and mastery were achieved after 25 and 40 cases, respectively.[34] Yet this data must be reviewed cautiously because learning curves are variable and more endoscopists with varying degrees of experience are needed to better define outcomes that extend beyond procedure times themselves.[35]

Technical Considerations

In terms of technique, EUS-GE can be carried out via a direct approach, EUS-guided double balloon-occluded gastrojejunostomy bypass (EPASS), or a wire-assisted technique.[4,5,36,37] There is no standardization yet but each procedure has distinct advantages and disadvantages to consider that have been analyzed in a recent meta-analysis.[38] All methods use a LAMS with a therapeutic channel linear-array echoendoscope (oblique or forward viewing based on operator preference) under general anesthesia. The prerequisite for any technique is proximity of the small bowel (duodenum or jejunum) to the stomach (**Figs. 2–4**). Instillation of fluid to distend this small bowel can be achieved using varying techniques but most commonly is done via an oro-enteric catheter placed across the site of obstruction, which can be used to instill water tinged with methylene blue. This, if chosen, allows for confirmation with a 19-gauge needle puncture that the target is the small bowel and not inadvertently the transverse colon. In certain situations, the small bowel can be directly punctured with a 19-gauge needle and contrast injected to distinguish small bowel from colon.

1. In the direct technique, a free-hand puncture with a cautery-enhanced LAMS is then made into the small bowel allowing deployment of the stent. The direct approach is now the most widely used technique because the use of a guidewire may encourage the small bowel to be pushed away while advancing the stent instead of penetrating it, leading to misdeployment.[36] It is also faster without any differences in technical outcomes compared with other methods.[39]

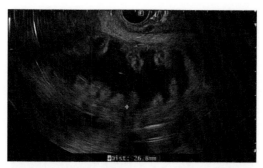

Fig. 2. Endoscopic ultrasound demonstrating the small bowel before needle puncture.

2. A balloon-assisted technique was the initial way an EUS-GE was performed. Over a guidewire, a dilating balloon or an endoscopic retrograde cholangiopancreatography (ERCP) extraction balloon is placed into the area of the small bowel to be targeted. This is punctured with a 19-gauge needle allowing access to the small bowel, and over this wire, a cautery-enhanced LAMS is deployed. In some situations, advancing the guidewire through the 19-gauge needle can be trapped in the targeted balloon and pulled out of the mouth (balloon traction method) to provide the safety of the distal end of the wire being secured. However, as mentioned above, this does not guarantee not misdeploying the prosthesis.

3. Initially described by Ito and colleagues in 2013, EPASS is a dedicated device, specifically designed for EUS-GE. The device consists of a catheter with 2 balloons, 20 cm apart, that is inserted past the stricture and inflated to distend and stabilize the target small bowel site.[40] This isolated area is filled with dilute contrast and methylene blue to allow for safe, direct puncture and LAMS deployment between the 2 balloons. This variation of the direct approach requires multiple steps and endoscopes, and a device currently not available in most countries but may ensure better fixation and distention of the small bowel for stent deployment.

Contraindications and Adverse Events to Endoscopic Ultrasound-Guided Gastroenterostomy

To date, contraindications are primarily based on expert opinion. In general, not being able to identify a targeted loop of bowel within 1 cm from the gastric wall or a small bowel obstruction downstream should preclude treatment.[37] The presence of minimal ascites typically should not be problematic; however, large volume ascites not

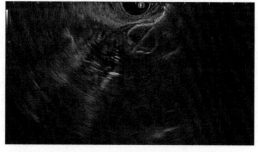

Fig. 3. Endoscopic ultrasound view of a jejunal flange deployed.

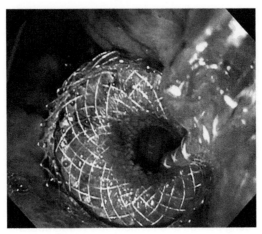

Fig. 4. Endoscopic view of a gastric flange deployed.

managed appropriately could lead to leaks, infection, and possibly interfere with tract maturation. Adverse events related to the procedure are most commonly due to stent misdeployment (typically the distal flange) leading to perforation. Postprocedure pain is rare given stent expansion is away from any malignant stricture as is bleeding due to the tamponading effect as the stent expands.[37] Stent misdeployment can be salvaged endoscopically in most cases with several techniques having been described.[41–43] A recent meta-analysis of 12 studies with 285 patients reported an adverse event rate of 12%.[44] Although this is already a low and acceptable number, it is likely that increased operator use and improvement in equipment and simplified techniques will lead to even lower numbers in the near future.

Endoscopic Ultrasound-Guided Gastroenterostomy Study Outcomes

EUS-GE has demonstrated excellent technical and clinical outcomes beyond 90% with limited adverse events that seem to decrease with increased operator experience.[45–48] A recent meta-analysis of 513 patients comparing EUS-GE, ES, and SGJ found that EUS-GE was associated with higher clinical success with lower rates of adverse events, reintervention, stent obstruction, and hospital stays.[49] In a study of 57 patients undergoing a direct EUS-GE approach for benign and malignant causes of GOO, clinical success was achieved in 89.5% of patients with only 2 adverse events over a median follow-up of 196 and 319.5 days for malignant and benign cases, respectively.[45] Furthermore, the median time to resuming a PO diet was only 1 day. During this extended period, the reintervention rate was 15.1%, with the majority of those (62.5%) unrelated to stent obstruction. A recent comparative study exploring long-term outcomes of EUS-GE was conducted at 2 centers with 436 patients (232 EUS-GE, 131 ES, and 73 SGJ) during a median follow-up time of 185.5 days (interquartile range 55.2–454.2).[48] The EUS-GE group demonstrated significantly higher rates of clinical success compared with ES and SGJ (98.3% vs 91.6% vs 90.4%), shorter median LOS (2 vs 3 vs 5 days), and lower rates of reintervention (0.9% vs 12.2% vs 13.7%).[48] Of note, the surgical group had lower ECOG scores than the EUS-GE and ES cohorts with lower rates of ascites and peritoneal carcinomatosis as well.[48] These studies highlight the advantage of EUS-GE in critically ill patients.

In addition to these advantages, a recent prospective study in Spain of 64 patients undergoing EUS-GE for malignant GOO revealed that there was a clinically significant increase (21.6 points on the global health status scale) in quality of life measures following the intervention.[50] Five other comparative studies between EUS-GE and SGJ have been conducted between 2017 and 2022 (**Table 1**).[51–55] Regardless of an open or laparoscopic approach, these studies have reinforced the clinical outcomes of EUS-GE with lower adverse events, decreased hospitalizations, and faster resumption of PO intake. In comparison to ES, a recent international propensity score analysis showed that EUS-GE was associated with a significantly higher clinical success (91% vs 71%) and lower rates of stent dysfunction (1% vs 26%).[56] Additional advantages over ES were found in a single-center study of patients with (n = 13) or without (n = 15) prior ES undergoing EUS-GE for malignant GOO in which the authors showed that EUS-GE as first line may limit repeat ES-related interventions and adverse events without disrupting chemotherapy treatment.[57]

The presence of ascites can be a limiting factor for SGJ. There is growing evidence that EUS-GE can be safely carried out in patients with ascites without major differences in technical outcomes, clinical success, and procedure times.[58] A recent single-center study of 55 patients (22 with small and 2 with large volume ascites) also found no major differences in clinical success, procedure time, and reintervention rates; however, there was a numerically higher adverse event rate (37.5% vs 19.4%) in those with ascites.[59] Sepsis and peritonitis were seen in 4 patients with ascites despite adequate periprocedural antibiotics. There also seemed to be a lower median survival in the ascites group (129 vs 180 days), which is more likely due to those patients having more advanced peritoneal disease. Yet the presence of ascites is not an absolute contraindication to EUS-GE. A therapeutic paracentesis can be performed first to allow for maximal drainage that may improve clinical outcomes. Considerations for a longer duration of antibiotic therapy could be considered.[60]

Finally, improvements in dedicated EUS-GE tools will continue to enhance outcomes. Notably, the availability of 20-mm LAMS can improve clinical outcomes, allowing a more liberalized diet.[52,61,62] A large multicenter study of 267 patients at 19 centers undergoing EUS-GE with a 15-mm (n = 148) and 20-mm (n = 119) for malignant GOO found that while technical, clinical, and adverse events did not differ, rates of reintervention (8.1% vs 4.2%) and toleration of a soft/complete diet at follow-up (81.2% vs 91.2%) favored the 20-mm LAMS.[61] Preliminary studies suggest that there seems to be no technical difficulties with an increased 20-mm flange, which is what we favor in our practice.

Endoscopic Ultrasound-Guided Gastroenterostomy Double Bypass

Another added benefit with EUS-GE is that simultaneous hepatic biliary drainage can be performed in patients with concomitant duodenal and biliary obstruction.[63–67] Our group recently published a case series of 23 patients undergoing single-session hepaticogastrostomy and gastrojejunostomy with a technical success rate of 100% and 95.6%, respectively.[64] Another analysis of 93 patients with biliary and duodenal obstruction undergoing various endoscopic approaches found that the combination of EUS-guided choledochoduodenostomy and ES were independent risk factors for frequent stent dysfunction.[67] Alternatively, combining biliary drainage with EUS-GE produced better outcomes with improved stent patency.

Management of Benign Gastric Outlet Obstruction

Balloon dilation

Endoscopic balloon dilation (EBD) is a well-established technique for treating benign causes of GOO.[68–70] A through-the-scope controlled radial expansion balloon dilator

Table 1
Studies comparing endoscopic ultrasound-guided gastroenterostomy versus surgical gastrojejunostomy for gastric outlet obstruction

First Author, Year	Study Design and Country	Number of EUS-GE vs SGJ	Technical Success (EUS-GE vs SGJ)	Clinical Success (EUS-GE vs SGJ)	Overall Adverse Events (EUS-GE vs SGJ)	Length of Hospital Stay, Days (EUS-GE vs SGJ)	Rate of Reintervention (EUS-GE vs SGJ)
Jaruvongvanich et al,[48] 2023	Multicenter, retrospective, Belgium and United States	222 vs 73	98.9% vs 100% (P = .58)	98.3% vs 90.4% (P<.0001)	8.6% vs 27.4%, (P<.0001)	2 vs 5 (P<.0001)	0.9% vs 13.7% (P<.0001)
Abbas et al,[51] 2022	Single center, retrospective, United States	25 vs 27	100% vs 100%, (P > .99)	88% vs 85% (P > .99)	8% vs 41% (P = .01)	25 vs 27	—
Bronswijk et al,[52] 2021	Multicenter, retrospective, Belgium, Netherlands, and United States	77 vs 48	94.6% vs 100% (P = .493)	97.1% vs 89.2% (P = .358)	2.7% vs 27% (P = .007)	4 vs 8 (P<.001)	—
Kouanda et al,[53] 2021	Single center, retrospective, United States	40 vs 26	92.5% vs 100% (P = .15)	85% vs 84% (P = .97)	2.25% vs 88%	5 vs 14.5 (P<.001)	20% vs 11.5% (P = .78)
Perez-Miranda et al,[54] 2017	Multicenter, retrospective, Spain, France, and United States	25 vs 29	88% vs 100% (P = .11)	84% vs 90% (P = .11)	12% vs 41% (P = .038)	9.4 vs 8.9 (P = .75)	—
Khashab et al,[55] 2017	Multicenter, retrospective, United States and Japan	30 vs 63	87% vs 100% (P = .009)	87% vs 90% (P = .18)	16% vs 25% (P = .3)	11.6 vs 12.2 (P = .35)	—

Abbreviations: EUS-GE, endoscopic ultrasound-guided gastroenterostomy; SGJ, surgical gastrojejunostomy.

can be used at various sizes based on the degree of narrowing with an endpoint of 15 mm over multiple sessions. The risk of perforation may increase with dilation greater than 15 mm. Clinical success is often defined by resolution in symptoms, traversability of the stricture and resolution of gastric residue. Strictures secondary to peptic ulcer disease have favorable long-term outcomes with 1 to 2 sessions of EBD and *H pylori* eradication.[69] However, strictures from caustic ingestion are exceedingly difficult to treat with refractory strictures occurring in up to 40% of cases.[71] Chronic pancreatitis can also be difficult to manage with one study reporting up to 5 EBD sessions without symptom resolution.[72] Refractory cases are often managed surgically.

Fully Covered Self-Expanding Metal Stent

To avoid surgery, endoscopic stenting is another option for refractory strictures. Alternatively, it may be used as a first-line option based on the degree of stenosis, location, and length. FCSEMS has been used in select cases, with early symptom improvement in more than 80% of individuals.[73–75] However, stent migration is a limiting factor, and despite suturing, can occur upward of 15% of cases.[73]

LAMS Across the Stricture

Similar to the off-label use of esophageal FCSEMS to treat benign strictures, LAMS have been placed for benign indications throughout the gastrointestinal tract, where one study reported limited migration rates over a median follow-up time of 301 days after stent placement.[76] In general, short (≤1.5 cm) benign strictures can successfully be treated with a LAMS placed across the stenosis. They have a lower migration rate compared with longer FCSEMS and are our stent of choice when managing short refractory benign gastroduodenal strictures.

Although the majority of EUS-GE studies have been for malignant cases, benign causes of GOO have been effectively managed with a technical and clinical success rate of 96.2% and 84%, respectively.[77] In patients who fail EBD, or is not technically feasible, and nor is a LAMS placement across the stricture, EUS-GE can be used. However, given that the standard of care is an SGJ (durable response and decades of data), consulting with the surgeons should be undertaken in a multidisciplinary approach before considering an EUS-GE. One single-center study of 22 patients found that 83.3% of patients were able to avoid surgery for definitive treatment, and only 5.6% developed recurrent GOO after EUS-GE.[78] An EUS-guided approach has also been used in several case reports in patients with super mesenteric artery (SMA) syndrome.[79–81] The stent dwell time depends if the underlying cause is reversible, such as resolution of pancreatitis, inflammation from other causes, and weight gain with SMA syndrome.

SUMMARY AND FUTURE CONSIDERATIONS

Endoscopic treatment of GOO continues to evolve with newer methods allowing for improved outcomes. The advent of therapeutic EUS has allowed for EUS-GE to emerge as a reliable and durable modality in patients with significant comorbidities and advanced disease who may not be ideal operative candidates. Development of novel devices (ie, cautery-enhanced LAMS) and refined techniques has allowed for technical success that rivals surgical and endoluminal stenting outcomes. Moving forward, prospective randomized trials comparing EUS-GE with ES and surgery have begun with results eagerly awaited.

CLINICS CARE POINTS

- For a new diagnosis of gastric outlet obstruction, in the absence of an obvious benign-appearing stricture, consider an endoscopic ultrasound to further elucidate the cause and rule out malignancy.
- If uncontrolled large volume ascites, consider using a duodenal stent over an EUS-gastroenterostomy.
- If the targeted loop of bowel is not within 1 cm from the gastric wall, then avoid an EUS gastroenterostomy.
- A 20-mm length stent should be preferred for an EUS GE.

DISCLOSURE

Dr S.S. Irani is a consultant for Boston Scientific, Conmed, and Gore. Dr A. Canakis declares no relevant funding for this study or financial relationships.

REFERENCES

1. Kumar A, Annamaraju P. Gastric Outlet Obstruction. In: StatPearls. StatPearls Publishing; 2022. Available at: http://www.ncbi.nlm.nih.gov/books/NBK557826/. Accessed January 27, 2023.
2. Tantillo K, Dym RJ, Chernyak V, et al. No way out: Causes of duodenal and gastric outlet obstruction. Clin Imaging 2020;65:37–46.
3. Tringali A, Giannetti A, Adler DG. Endoscopic management of gastric outlet obstruction disease. Ann Gastroenterol 2019;32(4):330–7.
4. Carbajo AY, Kahaleh M, Tyberg A. Clinical Review of EUS-guided Gastroenterostomy (EUS-GE). J Clin Gastroenterol 2020;54(1):1–7.
5. Irani S, Baron TH, Itoi T, et al. Endoscopic gastroenterostomy: techniques and review. Curr Opin Gastroenterol 2017;33(5):320–9.
6. Manuel-Vázquez A, Latorre-Fragua R, Ramiro-Pérez C, et al. Laparoscopic gastrojejunostomy for gastric outlet obstruction in patients with unresectable hepatopancreatobiliary cancers: A personal series and systematic review of the literature. World J Gastroenterol 2018;24(18):1978–88.
7. van Halsema EE, Rauws EA, Fockens P, et al. Self-expandable metal stents for malignant gastric outlet obstruction: A pooled analysis of prospective literature. World J Gastroenterol 2015;21(43):12468.
8. Espinel J, Sanz O, Vivas S, et al. Malignant gastrointestinal obstruction: endoscopic stenting versus surgical palliation. Surg Endosc 2006;20(7):1083–7.
9. Yoshida Y, Fukutomi A, Tanaka M, et al. Gastrojejunostomy versus duodenal stent placement for gastric outlet obstruction in patients with unresectable pancreatic cancer. Pancreatol 2017;17(6):983–9.
10. No JH, Kim SW, Lim CH, et al. Long-term outcome of palliative therapy for gastric outlet obstruction caused by unresectable gastric cancer in patients with good performance status: endoscopic stenting versus surgery. Gastrointest Endosc 2013;78(1):55–62.
11. Jeurnink SM, Steyerberg EW, van 't Hof G, et al. Gastrojejunostomy versus stent placement in patients with malignant gastric outlet obstruction: a comparison in 95 patients. J Surg Oncol 2007;96(5):389–96.

12. Canakis A, Baron TH. Therapeutic Endoscopic Ultrasound: Current Indications and Future Perspectives. GE Port J Gastroenterol 2023;1–15. https://doi.org/10.1159/000529089.

13. Ojima T, Nakamori M, Nakamura M, et al. Laparoscopic Gastrojejunostomy for Patients with Unresectable Gastric Cancer with Gastric Outlet Obstruction. J Gastrointest Surg 2017;21(8):1220–5.

14. Cheung SLH, Teoh AYB. Optimal Management of Gastric Outlet Obstruction in Unresectable Malignancies. Gut Liver 2022;16(2):190–7.

15. Al-Rashedy M, Dadibhai M, Shareif A, et al. Laparoscopic gastric bypass for gastric outlet obstruction is associated with smoother, faster recovery and shorter hospital stay compared with open surgery. J Hepatobiliary Pancreat Surg 2005; 12(6):474–8.

16. Zhang LP, Tabrizian P, Nguyen S, et al. Laparoscopic Gastrojejunostomy for the Treatment of Gastric Outlet Obstruction. J Soc Laparoendosc Surg 2011;15(2): 169–73.

17. Guzman EA, Dagis A, Bening L, et al. Laparoscopic gastrojejunostomy in patients with obstruction of the gastric outlet secondary to advanced malignancies. Am Surg 2009;75(2):129–32.

18. Jeong SJ, Lee J. Management of gastric outlet obstruction: Focusing on endoscopic approach. World J Gastrointest Pharmacol Ther 2020;11(2):8.

19. Hamada T, Hakuta R, Takahara N, et al. Covered versus uncovered metal stents for malignant gastric outlet obstruction: Systematic review and meta-analysis. Dig Endosc 2017;29(3):259–71.

20. Tringali A, Costa D, Anderloni A, et al. Covered versus uncovered metal stents for malignant gastric outlet obstruction: a systematic review and meta-analysis. Gastrointest Endosc 2020;92(6):1153–63.e9.

21. Pan Y min, Pan J, Guo LK, et al. Covered versus uncovered self-expandable metallic stents for palliation of malignant gastric outlet obstruction: a systematic review and meta-analysis. BMC Gastroenterol 2014;14:170.

22. Kim CG, Park SR, Choi IJ, et al. Effect of chemotherapy on the outcome of self-expandable metallic stents in gastric cancer patients with malignant outlet obstruction. Endoscopy 2012;44(9):807–12.

23. Kim JH, Song HY, Shin JH, et al. Metallic stent placement in the palliative treatment of malignant gastroduodenal obstructions: prospective evaluation of results and factors influencing outcome in 213 patients. Gastrointest Endosc 2007;66(2): 256–64.

24. Yamao K, Kitano M, Kayahara T, et al. Factors predicting through-the-scope gastroduodenal stenting outcomes in patients with gastric outlet obstruction: a large multicenter retrospective study in West Japan. Gastrointest Endosc 2016; 84(5):757–63.e6.

25. Grunwald D, Cohen J, Bartley A, et al. The location of obstruction predicts stent occlusion in malignant gastric outlet obstruction. Ther Adv Gastroenterol 2016; 9(6):815–22.

26. Jeon HH, Park CH, Park JC, et al. Carcinomatosis matters: clinical outcomes and prognostic factors for clinical success of stent placement in malignant gastric outlet obstruction. Surg Endosc 2014;28(3):988–95.

27. Hong J, Chen Y, Li J, et al. Comparison of gastrojejunostomy to endoscopic stenting for gastric outlet obstruction: An updated Systematic Review and Meta-analysis. Am J Surg 2022;223(6):1067–78.

28. Khamar J, Lee Y, Sachdeva A, et al. Gastrojejunostomy versus endoscopic stenting for the palliation of malignant gastric outlet obstruction: a systematic review and meta-analysis. Surg Endosc 2022. https://doi.org/10.1007/s00464-022-09572-5.

29. Roy A, Kim M, Christein J, et al. Stenting versus gastrojejunostomy for management of malignant gastric outlet obstruction: comparison of clinical outcomes and costs. Surg Endosc 2012;26(11):3114–9.

30. Jang S, Stevens T, Lopez R, et al. Superiority of Gastrojejunostomy Over Endoscopic Stenting for Palliation of Malignant Gastric Outlet Obstruction. Clin Gastroenterol Hepatol 2019;17(7):1295–302.e1.

31. Fritscher-Ravens A, Mosse CA, Mills TN, et al. A through-the-scope device for suturing and tissue approximation under EUS control. Gastrointest Endosc 2002; 56(5):737–42.

32. Binmoeller KF, Shah JN. Endoscopic ultrasound-guided gastroenterostomy using novel tools designed for transluminal therapy: a porcine study. Endoscopy 2012; 44(5):499–503.

33. Khashab MA, Kumbhari V, Grimm IS, et al. EUS-guided gastroenterostomy: the first U.S. clinical experience (with video). Gastrointest Endosc 2015;82(5):932–8.

34. Jovani M, Ichkhanian Y, Parsa N, et al. Assessment of the learning curve for EUS-guided gastroenterostomy for a single operator. Gastrointest Endosc 2021;93(5): 1088–93.

35. Perez-Miranda M. EUS-guided gastroenterostomy: closing knowledge gaps by evaluating learning curves. Gastrointest Endosc 2021;93(5):1094–6.

36. Irani S, Itoi T, Baron TH, et al. EUS-guided gastroenterostomy: techniques from East to West. VideoGIE 2019;5(2):48–50.

37. Law R, Irani S, Khashab MA. Endoscopic Ultrasound (EUS)-Guided Gastroenterostomy (EUS-GE). In: Testoni PA, Inoue H, Wallace MB, editors. Gastrointestinal and Pancreatico-biliary diseases: advanced Diagnostic and therapeutic endoscopy. New York City, USA: Springer International Publishing; 2020. p. 1–13. https://doi.org/10.1007/978-3-030-29964-4_55-1.

38. Ribas PHBV, De Moura DTH, Proença IM, et al. Endoscopic Ultrasound-Guided Gastroenterostomy for the Palliation of Gastric Outlet Obstruction (GOO): A Systematic Review and Meta-analysis of the Different Techniques. Cureus 2022; 14(11):e31526.

39. Chen YI, Kunda R, Storm AC, et al. EUS-guided gastroenterostomy: a multicenter study comparing the direct and balloon-assisted techniques. Gastrointest Endosc 2018;87(5):1215–21.

40. Itoi T, Itokawa F, Uraoka T, et al. Novel EUS-guided gastrojejunostomy technique using a new double-balloon enteric tube and lumen-apposing metal stent (with videos). Gastrointest Endosc 2013;78(6):934–9.

41. Sanchez-Ocana R, Penas-Herrero I, Gil-Simon P, et al. Natural orifice transluminal endoscopic surgery salvage of direct EUS-guided gastrojejunostomy. VideoGIE 2017;2(12):346–8.

42. Tyberg A, Saumoy M, Kahaleh M. Using NOTES to salvage a misdeployed lumen-apposing metal stent during an endoscopic ultrasound-guided gastroenterostomy. Endoscopy 2017;49(10):1007–8.

43. Abdelqader A, Nasr J. Natural Orifice Transluminal Endoscopic Salvage of Dislodged Endoscopic Ultrasound-Guided Jejunogastrostomy Stent After Endoscopic Retrograde in Roux-en-Y Anatomy. Am J Gastroenterol 2019;114(7):1024.

44. Iqbal U, Khara HS, Hu Y, et al. EUS-guided gastroenterostomy for the management of gastric outlet obstruction: A systematic review and meta-analysis. Endosc Ultrasound 2020;9(1):16–23.

45. Kerdsirichairat T, Irani S, Yang J, et al. Durability and long-term outcomes of direct EUS-guided gastroenterostomy using lumen-apposing metal stents for gastric outlet obstruction. Endosc Int Open 2019;7(2):E144–50.

46. McCarty TR, Garg R, Thompson CC, et al. Efficacy and safety of EUS-guided gastroenterostomy for benign and malignant gastric outlet obstruction: a systematic review and meta-analysis. Endosc Int Open 2019;7(11):E1474–82.

47. Tyberg A, Perez-Miranda M, Sanchez-Ocaña R, et al. Endoscopic ultrasound-guided gastrojejunostomy with a lumen-apposing metal stent: a multicenter, international experience. Endosc Int Open 2016;4(3):E276–81.

48. Jaruvongvanich V, Mahmoud T, Abu Dayyeh BK, et al. Endoscopic ultrasound-guided gastroenterostomy for the management of gastric outlet obstruction: A large comparative study with long-term follow-up. Endosc Int Open 2023;11(1): E60–6.

49. Boghossian MB, Funari MP, De Moura DTH, et al. EUS-guided gastroenterostomy versus duodenal stent placement and surgical gastrojejunostomy for the palliation of malignant gastric outlet obstruction: a systematic review and meta-analysis. Langenbeck's Arch Surg 2021;406(6):1803–17.

50. Garcia-Alonso FJ, Chavarria C, Subtil JC, et al. Prospective multicenter assessment of the impact of EUS-guided gastroenterostomy on patient quality of life in unresectable malignant gastric outlet obstruction. Gastrointest Endosc 2023; 0(0). https://doi.org/10.1016/j.gie.2023.02.015.

51. Abbas A, Dolan RD, Bazarbashi AN, et al. Endoscopic ultrasound-guided gastroenterostomy versus surgical gastrojejunostomy for the palliation of gastric outlet obstruction in patients with peritoneal carcinomatosis. Endoscopy 2022;54(7): 671–9.

52. Bronswijk M, Vanella G, van Malenstein H, et al. Laparoscopic versus EUS-guided gastroenterostomy for gastric outlet obstruction: an international multicenter propensity score-matched comparison (with video). Gastrointest Endosc 2021;94(3):526–36.e2.

53. Kouanda A, Binmoeller K, Hamerski C, et al. Endoscopic ultrasound-guided gastroenterostomy versus open surgical gastrojejunostomy: clinical outcomes and cost effectiveness analysis. Surg Endosc 2021;35(12):7058–67.

54. Perez-Miranda M, Tyberg A, Poletto D, et al. EUS-guided Gastrojejunostomy Versus Laparoscopic Gastrojejunostomy: An International Collaborative Study. J Clin Gastroenterol 2017;51(10):896–9.

55. Khashab MA, Bukhari M, Baron TH, et al. International multicenter comparative trial of endoscopic ultrasonography-guided gastroenterostomy versus surgical gastrojejunostomy for the treatment of malignant gastric outlet obstruction. Endosc Int Open 2017;5(4):E275–81.

56. van Wanrooij RLJ, Vanella G, Bronswijk M, et al. Endoscopic ultrasound-guided gastroenterostomy versus duodenal stenting for malignant gastric outlet obstruction: an international, multicenter, propensity score-matched comparison. Endoscopy 2022;54(11):1023–31.

57. Perez-Cuadrado-Robles E, Alric H, Aidibi A, et al. EUS-Guided Gastroenterostomy in Malignant Gastric Outlet Obstruction: A Comparative Study between First- and Second-Line Approaches after Enteral Stent Placement. Cancers 2022;14(22):5516.

58. Basha J, Lakhtakia S, Yarlagadda R, et al. Gastric outlet obstruction with ascites: EUS-guided gastro-enterostomy is feasible. Endosc Int Open 2021;9(12):E1918–23.

59. Mahmoud T, Storm AC, Law RJ, et al. Efficacy and safety of endoscopic ultrasound-guided gastrojejunostomy in patients with malignant gastric outlet obstruction and ascites. Endosc Int Open 2022;10(5):E670–8.

60. Bronswijk M, van Wanrooij RLJ, Vanella G, et al. EUS-guided gastroenterostomy in patients with ascites: What lies beneath? Endosc Int Open 2022;10(4):E294.

61. Bejjani M, Ghandour B, Subtil JC, et al. Clinical and technical outcomes of patients undergoing endoscopic ultrasound-guided gastroenterostomy using 20-mm vs. 15-mm lumen-apposing metal stents. Endoscopy 2022;54(7):680–7.

62. Madanat L, Saumoy M, Sharaiha RZ. Endoscopic gastrojejunostomy - bigger is better. Endoscopy 2018;50(12):E331–2.

63. Brewer Gutierrez OI, Nieto J, Irani S, et al. Double endoscopic bypass for gastric outlet obstruction and biliary obstruction. Endosc Int Open 2017;5(9):E893–9.

64. Canakis A, Hathorn KE, Irani SS, et al. Single session endoscopic ultrasound-guided double bypass (hepaticogastrostomy and gastrojejunostomy) for concomitant duodenal and biliary obstruction: A case series. J Hepatobiliary Pancreat Sci 2022;29(8):941–9.

65. Qatomah A, Nawawi A, Bessissow A, et al. Endoscopic ultrasound-guided gastrojejunostomy and choledochoduodenostomy with lumen-apposing metal stents: an efficient approach to double endoscopic bypass. Endoscopy 2022;54(S 02):E886–7.

66. Kongkam P, Luangsukrerk T, Harinwan K, et al. Combination of endoscopic-ultrasound guided choledochoduodenostomy and gastrojejunostomy resolving combined distal biliary and duodenal obstruction. Endoscopy 2021;53(9):E355–6.

67. Vanella G, Bronswijk M, van Wanrooij RL, et al. Combined endoscopic mAnagement of BiliaRy and gastrIc OutLET obstruction (CABRIOLET Study): A multicenter retrospective analysis. DEN Open 2023;3(1):e132.

68. Rana SS, Bhasin DK, Chandail VS, et al. Endoscopic balloon dilatation without fluoroscopy for treating gastric outlet obstruction because of benign etiologies. Surg Endosc 2011;25(5):1579–84.

69. Cherian PT, Cherian S, Singh P. Long-term follow-up of patients with gastric outlet obstruction related to peptic ulcer disease treated with endoscopic balloon dilatation and drug therapy. Gastrointest Endosc 2007;66(3):491–7.

70. Benjamin SB, Glass RL, Cattau EL, et al. Preliminary experience with balloon dilation of the pylorus. Gastrointest Endosc 1984;30(2):93–5.

71. Kochhar R, Malik S, Gupta P, et al. Etiological spectrum and response to endoscopic balloon dilation in patients with benign gastric outlet obstruction. Gastrointest Endosc 2018;88(6):899–908.

72. Kochhar R, Sethy PK, Nagi B, et al. Endoscopic balloon dilatation of benign gastric outlet obstruction. J Gastroenterol Hepatol 2004;19(4):418–22.

73. Randhawa NK, Khalyfa A, Khan M, et al. Safety and Efficacy of Fully Covered Self-Expandable Metal Stents for Benign Upper Gastrointestinal Strictures Beyond the Esophagus. Cureus 2022;14(11):e31439.

74. Choi WJ, Park JJ, Park J, et al. Effects of the Temporary Placement of a Self-Expandable Metallic Stent in Benign Pyloric Stenosis. Gut Liver 2013;7(4):417–22.

75. Heo J, Jung MK. Safety and efficacy of a partially covered self-expandable metal stent in benign pyloric obstruction. World J Gastroenterol WJG 2014;20(44):16721–5.

76. Irani S, Jalaj S, Ross A, et al. Use of a lumen-apposing metal stent to treat GI strictures (with videos). Gastrointest Endosc 2017;85(6):1285–9.

77. Chen YI, James TW, Agarwal A, et al. EUS-guided gastroenterostomy in management of benign gastric outlet obstruction. Endosc Int Open 2018;6(3):E363–9.
78. James TW, Greenberg S, Grimm IS, et al. EUS-guided gastroenteric anastomosis as a bridge to definitive treatment in benign gastric outlet obstruction. Gastrointest Endosc 2020;91(3):537–42.
79. Kouanda A, Watson R, Binmoeller KF, et al. EUS-guided gastroenterostomy for duodenal obstruction secondary to superior mesenteric artery syndrome. VideoGIE 2021;6(1):14–5.
80. Xu MM, Dawod E, Gaidhane M, et al. Reverse Endoscopic Ultrasound-Guided Gastrojejunostomy for the Treatment of Superior Mesenteric Artery Syndrome: A New Concept. Clin Endosc 2020;53(1):94–6.
81. Storm AC, Mahmoud T, Akiki K, et al. Endoscopic Ultrasound-Guided Gastrojejunostomy for Superior Mesenteric Artery Syndrome Secondary to Rapid Weight Loss. ACG Case Rep J 2022;9(10):e00868.

Endoscopic Management of Malignant Biliary Obstruction

Woo Hyun Paik, MD, PhD[a], Do Hyun Park, MD, PhD[b],*

KEYWORDS

- Biliary stricture • Jaundice • Malignant biliary obstruction • Endoscopic ultrasound
- Endoscopic retrograde cholangiopancreatography
- Percutaneous transhepatic biliary drainage

KEY POINTS

- Pros and cons of endoscopic retrograde cholangiopancreatography, percutaneous, and endoscopic ultrasound approaches for the management of malignant biliary obstruction.
- Factors to be considered when selecting the appropriate method of biliary drainage.
- Future direction in the management of malignant biliary obstruction.

Video content accompanies this article at http://www.giendo.theclinics.com.

INTRODUCTION

The primary carcinomas that cause malignant biliary obstruction (MBO) are periampullary tumors and perihilar tumors.[1–4]Video 1 However, MBO can also be caused by lymph node metastasis of other carcinomas, liver or peribiliary metastasis, and hemobilia accompanied by bile duct invasion of hepatocellular carcinoma.[5] Cancers, such as pancreatic cancer, cholangiocarcinoma, and duodenal cancer, that present with biliary obstruction at the time of diagnosis have a poorer prognosis than other solid cancers. Furthermore, biliary obstruction due to lymph node metastasis and peribiliary metastasis usually occurs in advanced stages of underlying cancers, which reduces the likelihood of timely biliary drainage. However, with recent advancements in anticancer therapy, the survival rate of cancer patients with biliary obstruction has

[a] Department of Internal Medicine and Liver Research Institute, Seoul National University Hospital, Seoul National University College of Medicine, 101 Daehak-ro, Jongno-gu, Seoul 03080, Korea; [b] Division of Gastroenterology, Department of Internal Medicine, University of Ulsan College of Medicine, Asan Medical Center, 88, Olympic-ro 43-Gil, Songpa-gu, Seoul 05505, Korea
* Corresponding author.
E-mail address: dhpark@amc.seoul.kr

Gastrointest Endoscopy Clin N Am 34 (2024) 127–140
https://doi.org/10.1016/j.giec.2023.07.004
1052-5157/24/© 2023 Elsevier Inc. All rights reserved.
giendo.theclinics.com

increased. Therefore, it is essential to consider various treatments for MBO in every patient, even those with advanced cancer.[6]

As endoscopic oncologists, we aim to review the benefits and drawbacks of various approaches, including endoscopic retrograde cholangiopancreatography (ERCP), percutaneous, and endoscopic ultrasound (EUS), in MBO, along with the associated treatment outcomes (**Fig. 1**). Furthermore, the future directions in managing MBO will be discussed.

THERAPEUTIC OPTIONS
Endoscopic Retrograde Cholangiopancreatography

ERCP is widely recognized as the first-line standard treatment for MBO due to its robust and acceptable clinical outcomes and its ability to effectively and safely relieve biliary obstruction.[7–9] Furthermore, bile excretion into the duodenum is restored after the procedure, providing physiologic advantages. However, the procedure always carries a risk of acute pancreatitis. In cases where intrahepatic ducts are separated, effective drainage with ERCP becomes challenging, leading to an increased likelihood of acute cholangitis and liver abscesses.[10] Additionally, the stent, such as uncovered or fully covered metal stent for MBO, may become susceptible to tumor ingrowth, overgrowth, or stent migration, which reduces stent patency.[11] The biofilm formation in a fully covered metal stent due to duodenobiliary reflux may also cause sludge formation and repeated stent malfunction. The most significant disadvantage of ERCP is the inability to perform the procedure if the endoscope cannot access the ampulla of Vater, such as in patients with a surgically altered anatomy or duodenal obstruction.

Percutaneous Approach

Percutaneous transhepatic biliary drainage (PTBD) is an established rescue method when ERCP fails.[12–14] PTBD is a highly successful procedure that offers the advantage

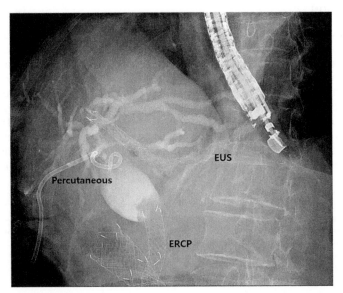

Fig. 1. ERCP, percutaneous, and EUS approaches in the management of malignant biliary obstruction. ERCP, endoscopic retrograde cholangiopancreatography; EUS, endoscopic ultrasound.

of being feasible even in cases where a patient's vital signs are unstable or a patient has a surgically altered anatomy. However, there are certain drawbacks to PTBD, including difficulty performing it when the patient has ascites, extensive liver metastases, or bleeding tendencies. Furthermore, tract seeding is risky if the catheter is carried out for an extended period.[15,16] Since the patient maintains the external drainage catheter, it can decrease the patient's quality of life and result in bile loss.[13] Internal stenting can be achieved through a percutaneous tract to mitigate the aforementioned drawbacks.[10] However, percutaneous or endoscopic reintervention will be challenging and cumbersome after internal stenting owing to the requirement of a new puncture for percutaneous biliary access or a different type of wire mesh in a percutaneously placed uncovered metal stent.

Endoscopic Ultrasound

EUS-guided biliary drainage (EUS-BD) is the most recent development among the 3 biliary drainage methods.[17–19] Its availability is currently limited to a few hospitals with the necessary resources to manage any EUS-BD–related potential complications involving an interventional radiologist or surgeon.[20] In cases where ERCP fails, the same endoscopist can perform EUS-BD immediately in the same session, and it has the advantage of draining bile inside the body, similar to ERCP.[21]

EUS-BD is a relatively new procedure and has not yet gained widespread popularity compared to ERCP.[22] Most of the published data on EUS-BD have been implemented by experts in EUS and ERCP. However, a significant advantage of EUS-BD over ERCP is that the stent patency period may be longer since the inserted stent bypasses the stricture rather than traversing the stricture as in ERCP.[11] Another advantage of EUS-BD is that it eliminates the risk of acute pancreatitis.[11] Therefore, it can be considered an initial treatment option for patients with a high risk of developing post-ERCP pancreatitis. Furthermore, EUS-BD can be a useful adjunct to PTBD and ERCP in cases where internal conversion of biliary drainage is required, or effective drainage is challenging due to separation of the intrahepatic duct (**Fig. 2**).[23,24] By clamping the PTBD tube for more than 24 hours, bile duct dilation can be induced. Moreover, the PTBD tube can facilitate cholangiogram by injecting contrast media through the tube, which enables the identification of the most suitable intrahepatic ducts for EUS-guided puncture. Additionally, even in cases of EUS-guided transhepatic biliary drainage (ETBD) failure, the burden on the operator appears to be minimal. Immediate declamping can facilitate bile duct decompression and minimize the risk of bile leakage.[14]

EUS-BD has various methods, such as transmural stenting, antegrade stenting, and rendezvous techniques, among which transmural stenting is a representative method.[25,26] Transmural stentings can be performed using two methods: an intrahepatic duct approach and a common bile duct approach. The intrahepatic duct approach seems to be more effective in addressing the limitations of ERCP or PTBD. A recently introduced term, ETBD, has been used to describe an approach to the intrahepatic duct equivalent to PTBD. Since the luminal access point with EUS can be from the esophagus, stomach, duodenum, or jejunum, ETBD may be a more appropriate term (**Fig. 3**, Video 1).[27,28]

The choice of stents for EUS-BD may be a prerequisite for successful EUS-BD in terms of preventing complications and enhancing clinical success, including stent patency. For EUS-guided hepaticogastrostomy (EUS-HGS), a partially covered tubular metal stent (intraductal uncovered portion) with a longer stent of 10 cm (especially braided-type stent) may be required to prevent fully covered stent-induced cholangitis by blocking the peripheral intrahepatic bile duct, and intraperitoneal stent

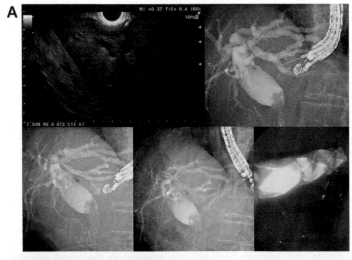

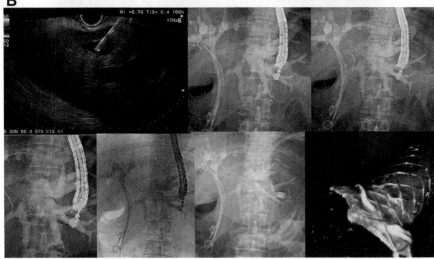

Fig. 2. Complementary biliary drainage using EUS in conjunction with (*A*) percutaneous or (*B*) ERCP approach. (*A*) Conversion of percutaneous transhepatic biliary drainage to EUS-guided transhepatic biliary drainage. (*B*) EUS-guided transhepatic biliary drainage of the left intrahepatic duct in combination with ERCP of the right intrahepatic duct is demonstrated for managing perihilar cholangiocarcinoma. ERCP, endoscopic retrograde cholangiopancreatography; EUS, endoscopic ultrasound.

migration by a long length of metal stent.[29] For EUS-guided hepaticoduodenostomy (EUS-HDS), intraperitoneal migration may not be common because the distance between the hepatic parenchyma in a left liver and stomach wall in EUS-HGS may be longer than that between hepatic parenchyma in a right liver and duodenum in EUS-HDS.[30] Therefore, less long stents, such as those 8 cm long, may be acceptable for EUS-HDS. If possible, stent revision could be required for EUS-HGS and HDS; a fully covered metal stent or dedicated plastic stent may be considered.[30]

In terms of EUS-guided choledochoduodenostomy (EUS-CDS), a tubular metal stent or lumen-apposing metal stent (LAMS) can be considered.[31–34] LAMS with

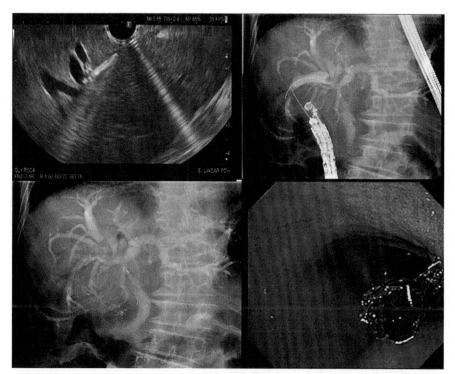

Fig. 3. EUS-guided transhepatic approach with diverse access points. (In a patient with gall-bladder cancer and common hepatic bile duct invasion, a transpapillary uncovered metal stent was placed in a left hepatic duct. After failed selective cannulation to the right intra-hepatic duct, EUS-guided hepaticoduodenostomy with a fully covered metal stent [6 mm in diameter and 8 cm in length] with antimigrating flaps was placed in the right posterior duct through EUS-guided hepaticoduodenostomy.) EUS, endoscopic ultrasound.

enhanced electrocautery may be preferred over tubular LAMS regarding technical convenience.[35,36] However, LAMS-related sump syndrome or food reflux may not be uncommon in patients with unresectable distal MBO and newly developed duodenal stenosis by pancreatic cancer progression during follow-up.[37–39]

SELECTION OF DRAINAGE METHODS

The selection of a bile duct drainage method should be based on consideration of the patient's condition and disease status, with various factors to be taken into account (**Table 1**). These factors include (1) the location of the biliary obstruction, (2) involvement of the cystic duct, (3) the degree of intrahepatic biliary dilation, (4) resectability, (5) the presence of liver metastases and ascites, (6) the presence of duodenal obstruction, (7) previous surgery history, and (8) the risk of bleeding.

For distal biliary obstruction, ERCP or EUS-BD is commonly used as a first-line treatment option. However, PTBD may be more effective for perihilar biliary obstruction. In cases where MBO involves the cystic duct, the risk of acute cholecystitis should be considered, especially with a fully covered self-expandable metal stent.[40] If acute cholecystitis occurs after ERCP, prompt management with biliary stent removal and antibiotics is necessary. If there is no improvement, EUS-guided or

Table 1
Comparison of ERCP, percutaneous, and EUS approaches for the management of malignant biliary obstruction

	ERCP	Percutaneous	EUS
Success rate	>90%	95%	>90%
Adverse events	Pancreatitis, cholecystit s	Bleeding, infection, dislodgement, tract seeding	Bile leak, bile peritonitis, stent intraperitoneal migration
Cause of dysfunction	Stent migration, sludge clogging, tumor ingrowth/overgrowth	Tube dislodgement	Food impaction, sludge clogging, stent migration
Advantage	Widely available Available in patients with non-dilated bile duct and bleeding tendency	Effective in advanced hilar obstruction	Free from pancreatitis Longer stent patency
Disadvantage	Less effective in advanced hilar obstruction Risk of pancreatitis	External drainage Most invasive Recurrent infection, tube dislodgement	Lack of data Safety issue Reimbursement issue
Limitation	Inaccessible papilla in patients with surgically altered anatomy or duodenal obstruct on	Multiple liver metastasis Ascites Bleeding tendency Non-dilated bile duct	Technical complexity Difficulty in training Bleeding tendency Non-dilated bile duct

Abbreviations: ERCP, endoscopic retrograde cholangiopancreatography; EUS, endoscopic ultrasound.

percutaneous cholecystostomy may be necessary. Recently, prophylactic EUS-guided gallbladder drainage for patients with MBO and cystic duct orifice involvement has been proposed.[41] Although the sample size of this study was too small, expanding the indication of EUS-guided gallbladder drainage may be considered for these highly selected patients.

When managing MBO, it is also essential to consider the extent of intrahepatic dilation. If the intrahepatic bile ducts are not sufficiently dilated, PTBD or ETBD may be technically challenging, and ERCP should be considered initially. Specifically, the intrahepatic duct must be dilated by at least 5 mm to facilitate successful ETBD.[42]

When planning for surgical resection in cases of MBO, ERCP or PTBD has been preferred over ETBD. This is because, during surgery, the stomach, which is commonly used as an access point for ETBD, may be manipulated, resulting in stent dislodgement. Pancreatitis is a common and potentially serious complication during ERCP before surgery.[43] As it may affect or delay the planned surgical procedure, special attention should be paid to minimize the risk of pancreatitis in these cases. Recently, EUS-CDS and conventional ERCP were compared regarding technical and clinical success, drainage-related complications, surgical complications, and oncological outcomes in patients requiring preoperative biliary drainage for distal MBO.[44] In this study, EUS-CDS was more efficient and associated with fewer surgical complications after pancreaticoduodenectomy without compromising the oncological outcome. However, further randomized control study on safety and efficacy of EUS-CDS and ERCP for patients with resectable distal MBO may be required to confirm these results. Before favorable results on EUS-CDS for resectable distal MBO are shown, primary EUS-CDS can be limitedly used for the treatment of unresectable distal MBO in real practice.

In patients with unresectable distal MBO, ERCP and EUS-BD can be equally considered when experts of both procedures are available. However, EUS-BD such as EUS-HGS or CDS may be preferred over ERCP in patients with surgically altered anatomy or duodenal obstruction when ERCP is unsuccessful or difficult ERCP is anticipated.[11]

In the case of perihilar biliary obstruction, ensuring drainage of the contralateral lobe is crucial, especially when right liver resection is necessary. In such cases, PTBD may be preferred to achieve sufficient drainage since the volume of the left liver is typically small.[15]

Managing MBO can be challenging in cases with multiple liver metastases, making it difficult to approach the bile duct by avoiding the metastasis. Consequently, PTBD or ETBD may be technically challenging in such cases. Additionally, in cases with ascites, the risk of bleeding after PTBD may increase, necessitating careful management.[45] Alternatively, EUS-BD may be a relatively safe approach, even in cases with ascites.[31,46]

As previously mentioned, if endoscopic access to the ampulla of Vater may be difficult due to duodenal obstruction or previous abdominal surgery, ETBD or PTBD may be considered as the first option. However, when the risk of bleeding is high, ERCP should be prioritized over ETBD or PTBD. This is because it is difficult to dilate the fistula tract with ETBD or PTBD under the risk of bleeding. In contrast, stent insertion via ERCP can be performed without an endoscopic sphincterotomy, thereby minimizing the risk of bleeding.

CLINICAL OUTCOMES
Efficacy

The success rate of the aforementioned 3 methods is more than 90%; however, each method may be difficult or less efficient in specific conditions, so clinicians should understand these situations well and choose optimal drainage methods for each situation.

When considering stent patency, ERCP involves passing the stent through a stricture, which carries the potential risk of stent ingrowth or overgrowth.[11] Furthermore, biofilm formation resulting from duodenobiliary reflux can lead to the recurrence of intrastent sludge, thus compromising stent function. Additionally, when managing external catheter maintenance during PTBD, there is a risk of inadvertent stent dislodgement. Considering all these factors, EUS-BD could provide the most favorable outcomes for stent patency. However, a potential risk of food impaction and stent migration warrants a head-to-head comparison of the biliary drainage methods in future studies.[47]

In economic terms, the cost-effectiveness of the 3 methods may vary slightly depending on the country. However, in general, ERCP is the most cost-effective option. Nonetheless, in the long run, EUS-BD with better stent patency and less reintervention might prove more cost-effective than ERCP, and further study is required to investigate this possibility.[48] In certain countries, reimbursement issues regarding EUS-BD need to be addressed.[28] Recently, a study analyzed the cost of PTBD and EUS-BD when performed as rescue therapy following ERCP failure.[49] The study combined biliary drainage costs and hospital stay costs, including the costs associated with treating adverse events, in Korea and the United States. The findings revealed that PTBD was associated with higher costs in both countries than EUS-BD, as reinterventions were more frequent in the PTBD group.

Safety

Although all 3 methods showed similar complication rates, the safety of EUS-BD is still debated due to limited available data, which are mainly published by experts.[50] In a recent meta-analysis, the rates of adverse events were similar between ERCP and EUS-BD (odds ratio 0.75, 95% confidence interval 0.45–1.24).[48] The types of adverse events, including bile peritonitis, bleeding, cholangitis, and cholecystitis, were similar between the 2 methods. Stent-related outcomes, including stent occlusion, stent migration, and stent dysfunction, were similar between the 2 methods.[48]

After ERCP failed, PTBD and EUS-BD showed similar success rates; however, the adverse events were fewer in EUS-BD.[51] In centers where EUS-BD is available, it may be a safer alternative to PTBD following a failed ERCP.[52]

Quality of Life

Theoretically, a better quality of life is expected with ERCP and EUS-BD than that with PTBD, as PTBD involves the inherent disadvantage of an indwelling external catheter. However, in a prospective study comparing EUS-BD and PTBD as primary biliary drainage methods, the difference in the quality of life was not statistically significant. This may be due to the high success rates of both procedures and the heterogeneity (internal stenting or external tube in place) of the PTBD group.[13] As survival rates for cancer patients continue to improve, there is a need for prospective studies to compare the quality of life outcomes of ERCP, EUS-BD, and PTBD.

COMPLICATIONS/CONCERNS

It is crucial to consider the potential complications of each of the 3 approaches and choose the safest method based on the individual situation. The most concerning and frequently encountered complication of ERCP is acute pancreatitis, which cannot be entirely prevented despite the use of rectal non-steroidal anti-inflammatory drugs and aggressive intravenous hydration.[53–55] Therefore, for patients with multiple risk factors for post-ERCP pancreatitis, considering EUS-BD as the first approach instead of ERCP may be appropriate, and prospective studies are necessary to establish its efficacy and safety. Patients at high risk of bleeding may find PTBD and ETBD challenging as the catheters or stents pass through the liver parenchyma, making ERCP a potentially safer option in such cases.

EUS-BD carries the risk of serious complications, such as bile leak resulting in bile peritonitis, intraperitoneal stent migration, pseudoaneurysm, and mediastinitis.[56–58] Therefore, it is crucial to carefully select appropriate patients for the procedure and have it performed by physicians with sufficient experience, with the backup of interventional radiologists and surgeons as needed to manage potential complications. Given the low rate of ERCP failure, next-generation ERCP performers may have limited experience with EUS-BD.[28] Whereas less than 1% of the cases in clinical practice require EUS-BD for naïve papilla,[59] mastering this technique requires approximately 100 cases to reach the learning curve plateau.[60] Therefore, training in EUS-BD is still challenging and requires a viable solution, including hands-on training or a simulator.

FUTURE DIRECTIONS

In the coming years, ETBD is poised to play an increasingly vital role as a less invasive and more quality-of-life-friendly alternative to PTBD. Conversion of external PTBD to ETBD can be a valuable technique for beginners in ETBD (see **Fig. 2**A).[28] To fully realize the potential benefits of ETBD, however, it is essential to develop safe and operator-friendly devices and accessories that can facilitate this technique.[61–65] When the intrahepatic duct is obstructed or separated, a combination of ERCP and ETBD may represent a promising strategy to prevent the occurrence of undrained bile ducts (see **Fig. 2**B). In patients with unresectable distal MBO, EUS-CDS with a LAMS may be a preferred first-line method over ERCP in terms of technical easiness. However, LAMS-related stent dysfunction with food reflux after EUS-CDS may not be uncommon in patients with the progression of duodenal stenosis during follow-up. Therefore, a better-refined technique of EUS-CDS with LAMS may be required for patients with unresectable distal MBO. As mentioned earlier, a prospective randomized trial comparing EUS-CDS with LAMS and ERCP for primary biliary decompression in patients with resectable distal MBO may be required to validate whether EUS-CDS with LAMS and ERCP may be equally effective for technical and clinical success and EUS-CDS with LAMS may be superior to ERCP in terms of postprocedural pancreatitis without compromising surgical and oncologic outcomes. By leveraging the complementary strengths of these techniques, this approach can help alleviate complications, such as cholangitis and biliary sepsis, and enhance treatment outcomes for patients with biliary obstruction.

SUMMARY

Managing MBO involves a range of options, including ERCP, PTBD, and EUS approaches, each with advantages and disadvantages. However, as new techniques and devices for ETBD continue to emerge, they are expected to become increasingly popular and replace PTBD. Nonetheless, it is important to note that ERCP, PTBD, and EUS each have unique strengths and limitations, and the choice of approach should be tailored to the individual patient's specific needs and circumstances.

CLINICS CARE POINTS

- The selection of bile duct drainage method for MBO should be based on the location of the obstruction, resectability, previous surgery history, the presence of duodenal obstruction, involvement of the cystic duct, the degree of intrahepatic biliary dilation, the presence of liver metastases and ascites, and the risk of bleeding.

- Although EUS-BD is available in limited hospitals with the necessary resources to manage any EUS-BD-related potential complications involving an intervention radiologist or surgeon, EUS-BD offers advantages in terms of stent patency compared to conventional ERCP or PTBD in the management of MBO.

- Unlike ERCP or PTBD, EUS-BD training is still challenging and requires a viable solution, including hands-on training or a simulator.

DISCLOSURE

D.H. Park is an inventor of an issued patent related to the Flap stent owned by Asan Foundation and MI-tech. The other author has no conflict of interest to disclose.

SUPPLEMENTARY DATA

Supplementary data related to this article can be found online at https://doi.org/10.1016/j.giec.2023.07.004.

REFERENCES

1. Razumilava N, Gores GJ. Cholangiocarcinoma. Lancet 2014;383:2168–79.
2. Cote GA, Sherman S. Endoscopic palliation of pancreatic cancer. Cancer J 2012; 18:584–90.
3. Valle JW, Kelley RK, Nervi B, et al. Biliary tract cancer. Lancet 2021;397:428–44.
4. Ryan DP, Hong TS, Bardeesy N. Pancreatic adenocarcinoma. N Engl J Med 2014;371:1039–49.
5. Chung KH, Lee SH, Park JM, et al. Self-expandable metallic stents vs. plastic stents for endoscopic biliary drainage in hepatocellular carcinoma. Endoscopy 2015;47:508–16.
6. Kang J, Lee SH, Choi JH, et al. Folfirinox chemotherapy prolongs stent patency in patients with malignant biliary obstruction due to unresectable pancreatic cancer. Hepatobiliary Pancreat Dis Int 2020;19:590–5.
7. Lokich JJ, Kane RA, Harrison DA, et al. Biliary tract obstruction secondary to cancer: management guidelines and selected literature review. J Clin Oncol 1987;5: 969–81.
8. Deviere J, Baize M, de Toeuf J, et al. Long-term follow-up of patients with hilar malignant stricture treated by endoscopic internal biliary drainage. Gastrointest Endosc 1988;34:95–101.
9. Stern N, Sturgess R. Endoscopic therapy in the management of malignant biliary obstruction. Eur J Surg Oncol 2008;34:313–7.
10. Paik WH, Park YS, Hwang JH, et al. Palliative treatment with self-expandable metallic stents in patients with advanced type III or IV hilar cholangiocarcinoma: a percutaneous versus endoscopic approach. Gastrointest Endosc 2009;69: 55–62.

11. Paik WH, Lee TH, Park DH, et al. EUS-Guided Biliary Drainage Versus ERCP for the Primary Palliation of Malignant Biliary Obstruction: A Multicenter Randomized Clinical Trial. Am J Gastroenterol 2018;113:987–97.

12. Glenn F, Evans JA, Mujahed Z, et al. Percutaneous transhepatic cholangiography. Ann Surg 1962;156:451–62.

13. Lee TH, Choi JH, Park do H, et al. Similar Efficacies of Endoscopic Ultrasound-guided Transmural and Percutaneous Drainage for Malignant Distal Biliary Obstruction. Clin Gastroenterol Hepatol 2016;14:1011–9.e3.

14. Paik WH, Lee NK, Nakai Y, et al. Conversion of external percutaneous transhepatic biliary drainage to endoscopic ultrasound-guided hepaticogastrostomy after failed standard internal stenting for malignant biliary obstruction. Endoscopy 2017;49:544–8.

15. Paik WH, Loganathan N, Hwang JH. Preoperative biliary drainage in hilar cholangiocarcinoma: When and how? World J Gastrointest Endosc 2014;6:68–73.

16. Son JH, Kim J, Lee SH, et al. The optimal duration of preoperative biliary drainage for periampullary tumors that cause severe obstructive jaundice. Am J Surg 2013; 206:40–6.

17. Giovannini M, Moutardier V, Pesenti C, et al. Endoscopic ultrasound-guided bilioduodenal anastomosis: a new technique for biliary drainage. Endoscopy 2001; 33:898–900.

18. Giovannini M, Dotti M, Bories E, et al. Hepaticogastrostomy by echo-endoscopy as a palliative treatment in a patient with metastatic biliary obstruction. Endoscopy 2003;35:1076–8.

19. Kim TH, Chon HK. [Endoscopic Ultrasound-guided Drainage in Pancreatobiliary Diseases]. Korean J Gastroenterol 2022;79:203–9.

20. Yamao K, Hara K, Mizuno N, et al. EUS-Guided Biliary Drainage. Gut Liver 2010; 4(Suppl 1):S67–75.

21. Han SY, Kim SO, So H, et al. EUS-guided biliary drainage versus ERCP for first-line palliation of malignant distal biliary obstruction: A systematic review and meta-analysis. Sci Rep 2019;9:16551.

22. Yoon WJ, Park DH, Choi JH, et al. The underutilization of EUS-guided biliary drainage: Perception of endoscopists in the East and West. Endosc Ultrasound 2019;8:188–93.

23. Park DH. Endoscopic ultrasound-guided biliary drainage of hilar biliary obstruction. J Hepatobiliary Pancreat Sci 2015;22:664–8.

24. Pal P, Lakhtakia S. Endoscopic ultrasound-guided intervention for inaccessible papilla in advanced malignant hilar biliary obstruction. Clin Endosc 2023;56: 143–54.

25. Paik WH, Park DH. Endoscopic Ultrasound-Guided Biliary Access, with Focus on Technique and Practical Tips. Clin Endosc 2017;50:104–11.

26. Bang JY, Hawes R, Varadarajulu S. Endoscopic biliary drainage for malignant distal biliary obstruction: Which is better - endoscopic retrograde cholangiopancreatography or endoscopic ultrasound? Dig Endosc 2022;34:317–24.

27. Hathorn KE, Canakis A, Baron TH. EUS-guided transhepatic biliary drainage: a large single-center U.S. experience. Gastrointest Endosc 2022;95:443–51.

28. Huh G, Park DH. EUS-guided transhepatic biliary drainage for next-generation ERCPists. Gastrointest Endosc 2022;95:452–4.

29. Cho DH, Lee SS, Oh D, et al. Long-term outcomes of a newly developed hybrid metal stent for EUS-guided biliary drainage (with videos). Gastrointest Endosc 2017;85:1067–75.

30. Ma KW, So H, Cho DH, et al. Durability and outcome of endoscopic ultrasound-guided hepaticoduodenostomy using a fully covered metal stent for segregated right intrahepatic duct dilatation. J Gastroenterol Hepatol 2020;35:1753–60.

31. Park DH, Koo JE, Oh J, et al. EUS-guided biliary drainage with one-step placement of a fully covered metal stent for malignant biliary obstruction: a prospective feasibility study. Am J Gastroenterol 2009;104:2168–74.

32. Bang JY, Varadarajulu S. Lumen-apposing metal stents for endoscopic ultrasonography-guided interventions. Dig Endosc 2019;31:619–26.

33. de Benito Sanz M, Nájera-Muñoz R, de la Serna-Higuera C, et al. Lumen apposing metal stents versus tubular self-expandable metal stents for endoscopic ultrasound-guided choledochoduodenostomy in malignant biliary obstruction. Surg Endosc 2021;35:6754–62.

34. Amato A, Sinagra E, Celsa C, et al. Efficacy of lumen-apposing metal stents or self-expandable metal stents for endoscopic ultrasound-guided choledochoduodenostomy: a systematic review and meta-analysis. Endoscopy 2021;53: 1037–47.

35. Tsuchiya T, Teoh AYB, Itoi T, et al. Long-term outcomes of EUS-guided choledochoduodenostomy using a lumen-apposing metal stent for malignant distal biliary obstruction: a prospective multicenter study. Gastrointest Endosc 2018;87: 1138–46.

36. On W, Paranandi B, Smith AM, et al. EUS-guided choledochoduodenostomy with electrocautery-enhanced lumen-apposing metal stents in patients with malignant distal biliary obstruction: multicenter collaboration from the United Kingdom and Ireland. Gastrointest Endosc 2022;95:432–42.

37. Geyl S, Redelsperger B, Yzet C, et al. Risk factors for stent dysfunction during long-term follow-up after EUS-guided biliary drainage using lumen-apposing metal stents: A prospective study. Endosc Ultrasound 2023;12(2):237–44.

38. Krishnamoorthi R, Dasari CS, Thoguluva Chandrasekar V, et al. Effectiveness and safety of EUS-guided choledochoduodenostomy using lumen-apposing metal stents (LAMS): a systematic review and meta-analysis. Surg Endosc 2020;34: 2866–77.

39. Paduano D, Facciorusso A, De Marco A, et al. Endoscopic Ultrasound Guided Biliary Drainage in Malignant Distal Biliary Obstruction. Cancers 2023;15(2):490.

40. Kim GH, Ryoo SK, Park JK, et al. Risk Factors for Pancreatitis and Cholecystitis after Endoscopic Biliary Stenting in Patients with Malignant Extrahepatic Bile Duct Obstruction. Clin Endosc 2019;52:598–605.

41. Robles-Medranda C, Oleas R, Puga-Tejada M, et al. Prophylactic EUS-guided gallbladder drainage prevents acute cholecystitis in patients with malignant biliary obstruction and cystic duct orifice involvement: a randomized trial (with video). Gastrointest Endosc 2023;97:445–53.

42. Oh D, Park DH, Song TJ, et al. Optimal biliary access point and learning curve for endoscopic ultrasound-guided hepaticogastrostomy with transmural stenting. Therap Adv Gastroenterol 2017;10:42–53.

43. Itoi T, Dhir V, Moon JH. EUS-guided biliary drainage: moving into a new era of biliary drainage. Gastrointest Endosc 2017;85:915–7.

44. Janet J, Albouys J, Napoleon B, et al. Pancreatoduodenectomy Following Preoperative Biliary Drainage Using Endoscopic Ultrasound-Guided Choledochoduodenostomy Versus a Transpapillary Stent: A Multicenter Comparative Cohort Study of the ACHBT-FRENCH-SFED Intergroup. Ann Surg Oncol 2023;30(8): 5036–46.

45. Ring EJ, Kerlan RK Jr. Interventional biliary radiology. AJR Am J Roentgenol 1984;142:31–4.
46. Alvarez-Sanchez MV, Luna OB, Oria I, et al. Feasibility and Safety of Endoscopic Ultrasound-Guided Biliary Drainage (EUS-BD) for Malignant Biliary Obstruction Associated with Ascites: Results of a Pilot Study. J Gastrointest Surg 2018;22: 1213–20.
47. Zhang HC, Tamil M, Kukreja K, et al. Review of Simultaneous Double Stenting Using Endoscopic Ultrasound-Guided Biliary Drainage Techniques in Combined Gastric Outlet and Biliary Obstructions. Clin Endosc 2020;53:167–75.
48. Lyu Y, Li T, Cheng Y, et al. Endoscopic ultrasound-guided vs ERCP-guided biliary drainage for malignant biliary obstruction: A up-to-date meta-analysis and systematic review. Dig Liver Dis 2021;53:1247–53.
49. Yoon WJ, Shah ED, Lee TH, et al. Endoscopic Ultrasound-Guided Versus Percutaneous Transhepatic Biliary Drainage in Patients With Malignant Biliary Obstruction: Which Is the Optimal Cost-Saving Strategy After Failed ERCP? Front Oncol 2022;12:844083.
50. Park DH, Jang JW, Lee SS, et al. EUS-guided biliary drainage with transluminal stenting after failed ERCP: predictors of adverse events and long-term results. Gastrointest Endosc 2011;74:1276–84.
51. Facciorusso A, Mangiavillano B, Paduano D, et al. Methods for Drainage of Distal Malignant Biliary Obstruction after ERCP Failure: A Systematic Review and Network Meta-Analysis. Cancers 2022;14:3291.
52. Sharaiha RZ, Khan MA, Kamal F, et al. Efficacy and safety of EUS-guided biliary drainage in comparison with percutaneous biliary drainage when ERCP fails: a systematic review and meta-analysis. Gastrointest Endosc 2017;85:904–14.
53. Talukdar R. Complications of ERCP. Best Pract Res Clin Gastroenterol 2016;30: 793–805.
54. Elmunzer BJ, Scheiman JM, Lehman GA, et al. A randomized trial of rectal indomethacin to prevent post-ERCP pancreatitis. N Engl J Med 2012;366:1414–22.
55. Park CH, Paik WH, Park ET, et al. Aggressive intravenous hydration with lactated Ringer's solution for prevention of post-ERCP pancreatitis: a prospective randomized multicenter clinical trial. Endoscopy 2018;50:378–85.
56. Paik WH, Park DH, Choi JH, et al. Simplified fistula dilation technique and modified stent deployment maneuver for EUS-guided hepaticogastrostomy. World J Gastroenterol 2014;20:5051–9.
57. Vila JJ, Perez-Miranda M, Vazquez-Sequeiros E, et al. Initial experience with EUS-guided cholangiopancreatography for biliary and pancreatic duct drainage: a Spanish national survey. Gastrointest Endosc 2012;76:1133–41.
58. Paik WH, Park DH. Outcomes and limitations: EUS-guided hepaticogastrostomy. Endosc Ultrasound 2019;8:S44–9.
59. Holt BA, Hawes R, Hasan M, et al. Biliary drainage: role of EUS guidance. Gastrointest Endosc 2016;83:160–5.
60. Tyberg A, Mishra A, Cheung M, et al. Learning curve for EUS-guided biliary drainage: What have we learned? Endosc Ultrasound 2020;9:392–6.
61. Binmoeller KF, Shah J. A novel lumen-apposing stent for transluminal drainage of nonadherent extraintestinal fluid collections. Endoscopy 2011;43:337–42.
62. Kahaleh M, Artifon EL, Perez-Miranda M, et al. Endoscopic ultrasonography guided biliary drainage: summary of consortium meeting, 2011, Chicago. World J Gastroenterol 2013;19:1372–9.

63. Park DH, Lee TH, Paik WH, et al. Feasibility and safety of a novel dedicated device for one-step EUS-guided biliary drainage: A randomized trial. J Gastroenterol Hepatol 2015;30:1461–6.

64. Paik WH, Park DH. Is there any tip that makes performing EUS-guided drainage easier and safer? Endosc Int Open 2017;5:E985.

65. Mangiavillano B, Moon JH, Crinò SF, et al. Safety and efficacy of a novel electrocautery-enhanced lumen-apposing metal stent in interventional EUS procedures (with video). Gastrointest Endosc 2022;95:115–22.

Endoscopic Management of Colonic Obstruction

Ahmad F. Aboelezz, MD[a], Mohamed O. Othman, MD[b],*

KEYWORDS

- Benign colonic obstruction • Malignant colonic obstruction
- Acute colonic pseudo-obstruction • Self-expandable metal stent
- Self-expandable plastic stent

KEY POINTS

- Endoscopic interventions are increasingly used for various causes of colonic obstruction to minimize the need for emergency surgery.
- Endoscopic management of colonic obstruction is indicated either as a palliative procedure or as a bridge to surgery. Endoscopic decompression, balloon dilation, stent insertion, debulking, or even percutaneous intervention can be performed by experienced endoscopists.
- Adverse events of endoscopic interventions include bowel perforation, infarction, and shock.

INTRODUCTION

Large bowel obstruction (LBO) is a serious event that occurs in approximately 25% of all intestinal obstructions.[1] It is attributed to either benign, malignant, functional (pseudo-obstruction), or mechanical conditions.[2] Benign etiologies of colonic obstructions include colon volvulus, anastomotic strictures, radiation injury, ischemia, inflammatory processes such as Crohn's disease, diverticulitis, bezoars, and intussusception. Malignant colonic obstruction is the main etiology of LBO and occurs in up to 20% of patients with advanced colorectal cancer.[3–5] In addition, patients with metastatic cancer and locally advanced pelvic tumors can also present with LBO.

Historically, a two-stage surgical resection was performed for the management of acute colonic obstruction. This approach consists of diverting colostomy with resection of the primary tumor. The colostomy can then be reversed after 8 weeks.[6] On some occasions, one-stage resection and primary anastomosis are performed. Given

[a] Department of Internal Medicine, Gastroenterology and Hepatology Section, Faculty of Medicine, Tanta University, El Bahr Street, Tanta Qism 2, Tanta 1, Gharbia Governorate 31111, Egypt; [b] Department of Internal Medicine, Gastroenterology and Hepatology Section, Baylor College of Medicine, Gastroenterology Section at Baylor St Luke's Medical Center, 7200 Cambridge Street. Suite 8A, Houston, TX 77030, USA
* Corresponding author. 7200 Cambridge Avenue, Suite 8A, Houston, TX 77030.
E-mail address: Mohamed.othman@bcm.edu

Gastrointest Endoscopy Clin N Am 34 (2024) 141–153
https://doi.org/10.1016/j.giec.2023.09.011
1052-5157/24/© 2023 Elsevier Inc. All rights reserved.

the high mortality rates and poor eligibility for surgery, endoscopic intervention has emerged as an alternative for two-stage surgical resection.[7] This article discusses the role of endoscopy in the management of LBO.

BENIGN COLONIC OBSTRUCTION

Patients with benign obstruction can present acutely with an abrupt onset of abdominal pain and distension, as in cases of colonic volvulus, intussusception, obstructed hernia, and diverticulitis. However, progressive narrowing of the lumen can present subacutely with bowel habit changes as in cases of anastomotic strictures or extraluminal compression of the colon. The lumen of the right colon is wider than the left one, making symptoms more insidious except for ileocecal valve location, which presents acutely two with intussusception.[8]

LBO occurs mainly in the cecum, hepatic and splenic flexures, or rectosigmoid colon.[9] Sigmoid colon and cecum are the most common sites of colonic volvulus.[10] Patients can present with rapid development of nausea, vomiting, abdominal pain, abdominal distension, and obstipation as in cases of acute volvulus. Other associated symptoms such as bleeding per rectum, unintentional weight loss, or presentation for a long time should raise awareness with malignancy or malignant transformation.

Colonic Volvulus

Colonic volvulus is sequelae of bowel loop twisting around the site of mesenteric attachment resulting in bowel obstruction, venous congestion, and eventually arterial flow obstruction.[11,12] Location of volvulus can lead to a variable presentation. For example, sigmoid volvulus is commonly seen in elderly patients with medical or neuropsychiatric comorbidities who often receive psychotropic medications leading to chronic constipation and subsequently sigmoid volvulus. Cecal volvulus, on the other hand, occurs in younger females.[13] Previous reports described that the gravid uterus elongates the cecal mesentery, making it more prone to torsion during or immediately after delivery. In addition, women in their mid-50s may be prone to pelvic surgeries as hysterectomy resulting in postoperative adhesions which act as an axis for cecal rotation.[14,15] Untreated volvulus leads to bowel ischemia, perforation, sepsis, and potential death.[16]

Endoscopic detorsion/decompression

Flexible sigmoidoscopy is considered first-line therapy in the management of sigmoid volvulus. Gentle advancement of the scope through the apex of converging colon mucosa "whirl sign" allows detorsion of the twisted colonic segment. This enables visualization of the colonic mucosa to asses for tissue viability and the presence of potential complications.[16] Placement of decompression tube is usually advised to maintain the colon decompressed and maintain the reduction of the volvulus. High recurrence rate after endoscopic decompression necessitates elective or semi-elective surgical treatment. Moreover, operative management is indicated after failed endoscopic decompression or if the patient presented with bowel perforation, bowel infarction, peritonitis, or septic shock.[17] Unlike sigmoid volvulus in which endoscopic decompression is the first line of therapy, colonoscopy is not generally recommended for the treatment of cecal volvulus and surgical management is typically preferred.

Percutaneous endoscopic colostomy

For patients unfit for surgery, percutaneous endoscopic colostomy (PEC) as an endoscopic sigmoidopexy is considered an alternative treatment. Although this procedure has significant morbidities and mortalities, it can be used to fixate sigmoid colon to the abdominal wall and prevent bowel twisting.[18,19]

Benign Colonic Strictures

Benign colonic strictures can result from diverticular disease, inflammatory bowel disease such as Crohn's colitis, ischemic colitis, radiation-induced colopathy, and postoperative anastomotic strictures due to ischemia, leak, or hemorrhage at the suture line.[20] Diverticulitis can lead to colonic obstruction in about 10% of cases. The main stay of treatment for benign bowel strictures is endoscopic dilation, dilation with steroid injection, and placement of decompression tubes or endoscopic stenting.

Endoscopic dilatation or stricturoplasty

Endoscopic dilatation of benign colonic strictures is performed through either the scope balloon or rigid Savary dilators. Simultaneous steroid injection or electroincision with placement of a decompression tube or expandable stent may be used in recurrent strictures. Endoscopic dilatation is performed for several indications such as in postoperative anastomotic strictures, strictures from inflammatory bowel disease (as Crohn's disease), colopathy induced by nonsteroidal anti-inflammatory drugs, and, complicated diverticulitis.[21]

Endoscopic balloon dilatation of anastomotic strictures is generally successful in resolving simple benign strictures, but results vary in post-radiation therapy strictures or in postoperative anastomotic leak. Repeated balloon dilatation may be required if restenosis occurred.[22]

For *Crohn's* colonic strictures, endoscopic balloon dilatation is generally successful in fibrotic strictures less than 5 cm in length, strictures without penetrating fistula, and when the stricture is in a straight bowel lumen and not in angulated part of the colon.[23,24] Intrastricture steroid injection did not show added benefit for complex *Crohn's* colonic strictures. East and colleagues in a pilot study of 13 patients who underwent local steroid injection versus saline placebo found that local quadrantic injection of triamcinolone did not reduce the time to radiation or surgery after balloon dilation of Crohn's ileocolonic anastomotic strictures.[25]

Endoscopic stricturoplasty depends on endoscopist's experience to determine the extent of luminal patency after endotherapy.[26] It can be used in refractory cases, angulated strictures, and anorectal strictures. Endoscopic stricturoplasty is performed by needle knife electroincision or cauterization of the stricture to break down the fibrous tissue and can be performed in a radial, horizontal, or circumferential fashion.[26–28]

Endoscopic stenting

Endoscopic stent placement can effectively decompress benign colonic obstruction either as a primary nonsurgical management or as a bridge to surgery (BTS).[29] This allows the conversion from an emergency to an elective one-stage surgery due to the avoidance of temporary stoma. This approach minimizes morbidity and mortality rates in comparison to open surgery in obstructed colons. Furthermore, the preoperative preparation of the bowel increases the probability of a successful primary anastomosis due to safer resection and less probability of contamination.[30] However, re-obstruction, migration, and perforation are considered the main delayed adverse events of endoscopic stenting. Adverse events usually occur 7 days after stent insertion.[31] Thus, it is preferable to consider elective surgery within this period after stent deployment.

Self-expanding metal stents (SEMSs), self-expanding plastic stents (SEPSs), and biodegradable stents (BDSs) can be used according to endoscopist preference and availability. SEMS can be covered or uncovered. The use of uncovered stents is usually not recommended in benign obstruction due to tissue growth through the metal mesh denoting extreme difficulty in removing it later on. Thus, it can be included in selected patients, as in patients with refractory colorectal stricture based on individual basis. In spite of higher rate of migration, covered stents are usually used, as they are easily removed endoscopically. Stent covering prevents granulation tissue growth within the stent mesh, reducing the risk of impaction.[32]

Clinical response to endoscopic stenting varies according to indication. SEMS placement in short ileocolonic anastomotic stricture due to *Crohn's disease* seems to be highly effective and safe. In a large prospective single-center series that included 21 patients with short (≤6 cm) fibrostenotic strictures of the terminal ileum or ileocolonic anastomoses, a partially covered stent was used, and endoscopic removal was performed 7 days after. Apart from stent-related discomfort and asymptomatic stent migrations, there were no direct stent-related complications such as perforation, impaction, or bleeding.[33] On the contrary, recurrent episodes of *acute diverticulitis* resulting in fibrosis and diverticular-associated colonic strictures do not respond favorably to endoscopic dilation or stenting.[34,35] In a systematic review by Currie and colleagues which included 130 studies and 122 patients, the use of SEMS in diverticulitis-associated strictures (*n* = 40) had a variable efficacy, which ranged from 43% to 95%. Efficacy in this study was defined as successful colon decompression, allowing for a complete colonic decompression and a one-stage surgical intervention. The median time to operation in this analysis was 14 days. The avoidance of stoma was successful in 17/40 (43%) patients and complications occurred in 21/40 (52%) patients.[36]

SEPSs (Polyflex stents) are reported in esophageal strictures,[37] however, they have been used in the rectum and distal sigmoid for temporary treatment of colonic obstructions in some studies as well.[38]

BDSs have been used in refractory benign esophageal strictures.[39,40] They are manufactured from various synthetic polymers, as polylactide or polyglycolide, or co-polymers, as polydioxanone. Their degradation depends on their size and structure. In addition, temperature, pH, and the type of body tissue/fluid around them influence their degradation as well.[41,42] Dilatation with BDSs is slow and it allows stricture remodeling around the stent as well as lower complication rates. Added benefit from BDS is that there is no necessity for its removal, thus providing cost reduction and allowing further procedures if needed. It usually takes about 4 to 5 weeks to lose its radial force, and after 9 weeks, radial force decreases to 50%.[43] However, there are limited data regarding its usage in colonic strictures.

The lumen-apposing metal stent (LAMS) is a saddle-shaped stent with bilateral anchoring flanges that provide anti-migratory lumen apposing advantage. Originally, it was designed for pancreatic fluid collection drainage, but it showed a beneficial role in refractory benign colonic strictures. A LAMS can be placed across a stricture via either direct endoscopic visualization with or without fluoroscopic guidance or an endoscopic ultrasound (EUS)-guided approach. An observational, retrospective, single-arm, multicenter study of 30 patients undergoing LAMS placement for benign luminal gastrointestinal stricture, Yang and colleagues reported that LAMS placement demonstrated a safe, feasible, and effective therapeutic option for patients with benign luminal gastrointestinal strictures with a low stent migration rate as well.[44]

Transanal decompression tubes

Endoscopic transanal tube decompression is usually reserved for acute colonic obstruction. In a study by Fischer and colleagues, which identified 51 patients of acute colonic obstructions including 9 benign cases of different etiologies, endoscopic tube decompression for acute colonic obstructions, allowed the conversion from emergent to elective or semi-elective operation in 73% of patients. Therefore, a better quality of life and favorable social and personal outcomes were achieved.[45]

Acute Colonic Pseudo-Obstruction

Acute colonic pseudo-obstruction (ACPO), often referred to as Ogilvie syndrome, is a clinical condition characterized by severe distension of the large intestine without mechanical obstruction. It can result in serious adverse events such as abdominal ischemia and perforation if left untreated.[46] These adverse events are particularly noted in patients with cecal diameters greater than 10 to 12 cm and if the duration of distention is more than 6 days.[47]

It is crucial to exclude mechanical causes of colonic obstruction. Plain-film abdominal radiography showing massive colon dilation, often limited to the cecum and right colon, is the first clue of the ACPO.[48,49] Additional testing such as water-soluble contrast enema is performed not only as a diagnostic option but in the hope that it may be successful in decompressing ACPO.[50] However, CT has largely replaced contrast enema studies in the last two decades.

Conservative management through avoiding predisposing factors such as narcotics and correction of fluid and electrolyte imbalance is the first-line therapy of ACPO. Serial assessment of cecal diameter is crucial because of the high risk of colonic perforation. The persistence of symptoms for more than 48 to 72 hours necessitates neostigmine administration as a pharmacologic therapy or endoscopic intervention.[2]

Endoscopic decompression

Endoscopic decompression is performed using water infusion with or without minimal carbon dioxide insufflation rather than air. As previously mentioned, exclusion of perforation with a plain abdominal x-ray and clinical evaluation of patients especially in the presence of fever, leukocytosis, or worsening abdominal pain should be done before performing endoscopic decompression.[2] Sedation using benzodiazepines or other nonnarcotic medication is preferred over narcotics. The endoscopic decompression is challenging as it is performed in an unprepared colon. Cecal intubation is usually unnecessary; however, attempts to reach the distal transverse colon should be done with extensive air suctioning to depressurize the colon.[51,52] There is contradictory data about decompression tube insertion and whether it can decrease recurrence rate. However, polyethylene glycol solution after endoscopy could play a role in reducing recurrence.[53–55] The risk of perforation and mortality are 2% and 1%, respectively. In addition, there is a 40% risk of recurrence necessitating repeated colonoscopic decompression.[56]

Percutaneous endoscopic colostomy

PEC is an alternative endoscopic technique that is performed in patients who have failed to respond to pharmacologic or endoscopic decompression therapy. It is a minimally invasive procedure with a plastic tube placement into the cecum or left colon.[57,58] Tube insertion through endoscopic and radiologic approaches allows the irrigation and/or decompression with a success rates up to 100%.[58,59] However, adverse events including wound infection, bleeding, hematoma formation, perforation with subsequent peritonitis, granuloma, or buried bumper have been reported.[60]

MALIGNANT COLONIC OBSTRUCTION

Colorectal cancer is one of the most common cancers worldwide.[61] Unfortunately, in spite of active screening programs for colorectal cancer, partial or complete bowel obstruction remains a common initial presentation of the illness and its incidence has not changed.[62] Acute colonic obstruction complicates approximately 20% to 25% of patients with primary colorectal cancer.[63,64] Metastatic disease to the colon also may cause colonic obstruction, and extracolonic pelvic tumors may result in external colonic compression or colonic invasion with subsequent colonic obstruction.[65]

Most of the colonic adenocarcinomas causing obstruction are located in the left side of the colon with the sigmoid colon representing the single most common site of obstruction due to its narrow lumen.[66] However, the rectum is the least frequent location for colonic obstruction due to its sizable lumen and the associated alarming symptoms of bleeding and difficulty in defecation leading to early diagnosis of rectal cancer. On the contrary to the sigmoid colon, the cecum and ascending colon have a larger lumen making the tumor more bulky and more locally advanced than left-sided.[67,68] Endoscopic management of malignant colonic obstruction is generally similar to benign one with less emphasis on endoscopic dilation due to its ineffectiveness.

Endoscopic Tube Insertion for Decompression

Decompression tubes insertion are a temporary, relatively cheap, and widely available method to relieve colonic obstruction. However, it cannot be inserted permanently for palliation. In addition, it may cause patient discomfort and there is a risk of tube expulsion, bleeding, and perforation during insertion.[65] Transanal endoscopic placement of a tube with immediate colonic decompression may allow the patient to undergo a one-stage surgery without colostomy formation if it worked successfully.[69,70]

Self-Expandable Metal Stent

Colonic stents are inserted either through the scope (TTS) or non-TTS. Fluoroscopic guidance usually accompanies the endoscopic insertion of colonic stent. Colonic stents are either covered or uncovered. Covered stents have lower risk of tumor ingrowth, thus, they can be used for sealing fistulas. However, they have a higher risk of migration. On the other hand, uncovered stents carry a lower risk for migration, nevertheless, a higher tumor in growth rate.[71]

SEMS is a significantly less invasive procedure than emergency surgery and it allows the optimization of the patient's clinical state before the surgery, including a better nutritional status, prepared bowel, and corrected electrolyte disturbances.

SEMS as a bridge to surgery: Stenting is recommended by the European Society of Gastrointestinal Endoscopy as a BTS. Endoscopic stenting should be discussed, within a shared decision-making process, as a treatment option in patients with potentially curable left-sided obstructing colon cancer.[72] SEMS, as compared with emergency surgery, reduces the length of hospital stay, generates higher rates of successful primary colonic anastomosis, and minimizes the need for stoma formation, and lowers leak rates.[6,73,74] In addition, staging of the tumor can be evaluated, and this allows the administration of neoadjuvant therapy in patients with rectal cancer.[5] **Fig. 1** illustrates SEMS insertion as BTS in left-sided colonic tumor.

The time interval between SEMS insertion and surgery remains controversial. A retrospective study by Oh and colleagues ($n = 148$) showed a bridging interval of more than 2 weeks between SEMS insertion and surgery for left malignant colonic obstruction has favorable short-term clinical outcomes, lower rates of stoma formation, and higher rate of laparoscopic surgery.[75] Another large prospective, multicenter feasibility study by Saito and colleagues ($n = 297$) of SEMS as a bridge to therapy showed that the median time between SEMS and surgery was 16 days and a longer interval did not increase the incidence of anastomotic leakage or conversion from laparoscopic to open surgery.[76]

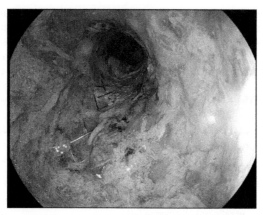

Fig. 1. SEMS insertion as bridge to surgery in left-sided colonic tumor.

SEMS for palliation: Palliative SEMS permits early nutrition, lower rates of stoma formation, reduced hospital stay, and better quality of life.[77] With regard to the location of stent insertion, a study done by Tal and colleagues compared the outcome of palliative noncovered SEMS placement in left-sided versus proximal colonic obstruction. The study showed a safe and effective palliation of malignant obstruction regardless of the location of the tumor in the colon.[78] Stent-related complications are perforation, stent migration, and obstruction.[79] In a retrospective multicenter cohort study, Siddiqui and colleagues found that maintenance of colonic decompression without the recurrence of bowel obstruction until patient death or last follow-up was lower in the SEMS group (73.9%) compared with surgery group (94.4%).[80]

SEMS for extracolonic compression: Extrinsic colonic obstruction most probably results from metastatic tumors to the pelvis, pelvic tumors (bladder, ovaries, or uterus), or small bowel tumors.[81] In a large retrospective series of colonic stent placement for LBO in extracolonic malignancy patients by Faraz and colleagues, technical and clinical success rates in this rare indication were 75.9% and 54.5%, respectively. Given disease burden, reduced life expectancy, and unfitness for surgery, SEMS are usually placed in extracolonic compression.[82]

Endoscopic Tumor Debulking

Patients who are unfit for surgery can be evaluated for tumor debulking through endoscopic laser therapy or argon plasma coagulation (APC).[83,84] Given that it is difficult to prepare the colon in the setting of intestinal obstruction, APC use is hindered due to the risk of colon explosion. In addition, its safety and effectiveness have been reported only in small case series.[84]

Endoscopic laser therapy may provide an effective relief of local symptoms such as bleeding, tenesmus, and mucus discharge from rectal carcinomas. Also, it allows intrinsic bulky tumor recanalization under direct vision. However, it is technically difficult above the sigmoid colon and is usually performed in rectal and left-sided colon.[85]

SUMMARY

Different endoscopic techniques have emerged in the recent years for LBOs. These procedures aim for a quick, safe, and effective management of the obstruction whether as a palliative therapy or BTS, thus avoiding emergent surgery. Early endoscopic interventions either through endoscopic decompression, dilation, stenting, or electro-incision decrease morbidity and mortality, improve nutritional status, and provide a better quality of life. In addition, it allows implementation of neoadjuvant therapy and evaluating the tumor stage in malignant cases. The decision for early endoscopic interventions in these setting should be considered in a multidisciplinary fashion.

CLINICS CARE POINTS

- Pearls Sigmoid colon is a common site for volvulus.
- The first line therapy for sigmoid volvulus is endoscopic detorsion.
- Insertion of decompression tube is the next step before considering surgical intervention.
- In case of cecal volvulus, surgical intervention is the typical management and colonoscopic decompression is generally not recommended.
- Simple Crohn's colonic strictures is usually less than 5 cm in length and located in a straight bowel lumen.
- Balloon dilatation is sufficient for managing these simple strictures.
- Stricturoplasty is reserved for refractory, angulated or anorectal strictures.
- Failed conservative management of acute colonic pseudo-obstruction "after 48-72 hours" necessitates either neostigmine administration or endoscopic decompression.
- Malignant colonic obstruction or extracolonic compression causing obstruction should be initially treated with self-expanding metal stent (SEMS).
- SEMS placement as bridge to surgery optimizes patients' clinical condition, avoids stoma creation and provide better surgical outcomes.
- SEMS could also be placed for palliative purposes in non-surgical patients.

CONFLICT OF INTEREST

M.O. Othman: M.O. Othman is a consultant for Olympus, Boston Scientific Corporation, Abbvie, ConMed, Neptune Medical, Creo Medical, Lumendi, and Apollo. MO Othman received research grants from Lucid Diagnostics, AbbVie, United States, Nestle, ConMed, United States, Olympus and Boston Scientific.

REFERENCES

1. Markogiannakis H, Messaris E, Dardamanis D, et al. Acute mechanical bowel obstruction: clinical presentation, etiology, management and outcome. World J Gastroenterol 2007;13(3):432–7.
2. Naveed M, Jamil LH, Fujii-Lau LL, et al. American Society for Gastrointestinal Endoscopy guideline on the role of endoscopy in the management of acute colonic pseudo-obstruction and colonic volvulus. Gastrointest Endosc 2020;91: 228–35.
3. Jemal A, Bray F, Center MM, et al. Global cancer statistics. CA Cancer J Clin 2011;61(2):69–90.
4. Seo SY, Kim SW. Endoscopic management of malignant colonic obstruction. Clin Endosc 2020;53(1):9.
5. Harrison M, Anderson M, Appalaneni V, et al. The role of endoscopy in the management of patients with known and suspected colonic obstruction and pseudo-obstruction. Gastrointest Endosc 2010. https://doi.org/10.1016/j.gie.2009.11.027.

6. Targownik LE, Spiegel BM, Sack J, et al. Colonic stent vs. emergency surgery for management of acute left-sided malignant colonic obstruction: a decision analysis. Gastrointest Endosc 2004;60(6):865–74.

7. Olson TJP, Pinkerton C, Brasel KJ, et al. Palliative surgery for malignant bowel obstruction from carcinomatosis: a systematic review. JAMA Surg 2014;149(4):383.

8. Taourel P, Kessler N, Lesnik A, Pujol J, Morcos L, Bruel JM. Helical CT of large bowel obstruction. Abdom Imaging. 2003;28(2):267-275. Accessed February 19, 2023. https://www.academia.edu/10061526/Helical_CT_of_large_bowel_obstruction

9. Cannella R, Taibbi A, Porrello G, et al. Hepatocellular carcinoma with macrovascular invasion: multimodality imaging features for the diagnosis. Diagnostic Interv Radiol 2020;26(6):531.

10. Ballantyne GH, Brandner MD, Beart RW, et al. Volvulus of the colon. Incidence and mortality. Ann Surg 1985;202(1):83.

11. Gingold D, Murrell Z. Management of colonic volvulus. Clin Colon Rectal Surg 2012;25(4):236.

12. Ballantyne GH, Brandner MD, Beart RW, et al. Volvulus of the colon incidence and mortality. Ann Surg 1985.

13. Halabi WJ, Jafari MD, Kang CY, et al. Colonic volvulus in the United States: Trends, outcomes, and predictors of mortality. Ann Surg 2014;259(2):293–301.

14. Pal A, Corbett E, Mahadevan N. Caecal volvulus secondary to malrotation presenting after caesarean section. J Obstet Gynaecol 2005;25(8):805–6.

15. Whiteman MK, Hillis SD, Jamieson DJ, et al. Inpatient hysterectomy surveillance in the United States, 2000-2004. Am J Obstet Gynecol 2008;198(1):34.e1–7.

16. jiang TS, Wu R. Endoscopic decompression, detorsion, and reduction of sigmoid volvulus. Video J Encycl GI Endosc 2014;2(1):20–5.

17. Labkin JO, Thekiso TB, Waldron R, et al. Recurrent sigmoid volvulus – early resection may obviate later emergency surgery and reduce morbidity and mortality. Ann R Coll Surg Engl 2009;91(3):205.

18. Tun G, Bullas D, Bannaga A, et al. Percutaneous endoscopic colostomy: a useful technique when surgery is not an option. Ann Gastroenterol Q Publ Hell Soc Gastroenterol 2016;29(4):477.

19. Baraza W, Brown S, McAlindon M, et al. Prospective analysis of percutaneous endoscopic colostomy at a tertiary referral centre. Br J Surg 2007;94(11):1415–20.

20. Liangpunsakul S, Rex DK. Management of benign colonic strictures. Tech Gastrointest Endosc 2003;5(4):178–81.

21. Ali SE, Bhakta A, Bautista RM, et al. Endoscopic stricturotomy with pulsed argon plasma and balloon dilation for refractory benign colorectal strictures: a case series. Transl Gastroenterol Hepatol 2022;7(0).

22. Chan RH, Lin SC, Chen PC, et al. Management of colorectal anastomotic stricture with multidiameter balloon dilation: long-term results. Tech Coloproctol 2020;24(12):1271.

23. Felley C, Vader JP, Juillerat P, et al. Appropriate therapy for fistulizing and fibrostenotic Crohn's disease: Results of a multidisciplinary expert panel - EPACT II. J Crohns Colitis 2009;3(4):250–6.

24. Paine E, Shen B. Endoscopic therapy in inflammatory bowel diseases (with videos). Gastrointest Endosc 2013;78(6):819–35.

25. East JE, Brooker JC, Rutter MD, et al. A pilot study of intrastricture steroid versus placebo injection after balloon dilatation of Crohn's strictures. Clin Gastroenterol Hepatol 2007;5(9):1065–9.

26. Shen B. Interventional IBD: the role of endoscopist in the multidisciplinary team management of IBD. Inflamm Bowel Dis 2018;24(2):298–309.
27. Shen B, Kochhar G, Navaneethan U, et al. Practical guidelines on endoscopic treatment for Crohn's disease strictures: a consensus statement from the Global Interventional Inflammatory Bowel Disease Group. lancet Gastroenterol Hepatol 2020;5(4):393–405.
28. Lan N, Shen B. Endoscopic stricturotomy with needle knife in the treatment of strictures from inflammatory bowel disease. Inflamm Bowel Dis 2017;23(4): 502–13.
29. Jovani M, Genco C, Bravatà I, et al. Stents in the management of benign colorectal strictures. Tech Gastrointest Endosc 2014;16(3):135–41.
30. Small AJ, Young-Fadok TM, Baron TH. Expandable metal stent placement for benign colorectal obstruction: Outcomes for 23 cases. Surg Endosc Other Interv Tech 2008;22(2):454–62.
31. Keränen I, Lepistö A, Udd M, et al. Outcome of patients after endoluminal stent placement for benign colorectal obstruction. Scand J Gastroenterol 2010;45(6): 725–31.
32. Hong JT, Kim TJ, Hong SN, et al. Uncovered self-expandable metal stents for the treatment of refractory benign colorectal anastomotic stricture. Sci Reports 2020; 10(1):1–9.
33. Das R, Singh R, Din S, et al. Therapeutic resolution of focal, predominantly anastomotic Crohn's disease strictures using removable stents: outcomes from a single-center case series in the United Kingdom. Gastrointest Endosc 2020; 92(2):344–52.
34. Fejleh MP, Tabibian JH. Colonoscopic management of diverticular disease. World J Gastrointest Endosc 2020;12(2):53–9.
35. Graham DY, Tabibian N, Schwartz JT, et al. Evaluation of the effectiveness of through-the-scope balloons as dilators of benign and malignant gastrointestinal strictures. Gastrointest Endosc 1987;33(6):432–5.
36. Currie A, Christmas C, Aldean H, et al. Systematic review of self-expanding stents in the management of benign colorectal obstruction. Colorectal Dis 2014. https://doi.org/10.1111/codi.12389.
37. Conio M, Repici A, Battaglia G, et al. A randomized prospective comparison of self-expandable plastic stents and partially covered self-expandable metal stents in the palliation of malignant esophageal dysphagia. Am J Gastroenterol 2007; 102(12):2667–77.
38. García-Cano J. Dilation of benign strictures in the esophagus and colon with the polyflex stent: a case series study. Dig Dis Sci 2007;53(2):341–6.
39. Fry SW, Fleischer DE. Management of a refractory benign esophageal stricture with a new biodegradable stent. Gastrointest Endosc 1997;45(2):179–82.
40. Stivaros SM, Williams LR, Senger C, et al. Woven polydioxanone biodegradable stents: a new treatment option for benign and malignant oesophageal strictures. Eur Radiol 2010;20(5):1069–72.
41. Freudenberg S, Rewerk S, Kaess M, et al. Biodegradation of absorbable sutures in body fluids and pH buffers. Eur Surg Res 2004;36(6):376–85.
42. Gunatillake P, Mayadunne R, Adhikari R. Recent developments in biodegradable synthetic polymers. Biotechnol Annu Rev 2006;12:301–47.
43. Rejchrt S, Kopacova M, Brozik J, et al. Biodegradable stents for the treatment of benign stenoses of the small and large intestines. Endoscopy 2011;43(10): 911–7.

44. Yang D, Nieto JM, Siddiqui A, et al. Lumen-apposing covered self-expandable metal stents for short benign gastrointestinal strictures: a multicenter study. Endoscopy 2017;49(4):327–33.
45. Fischer A, Schrag HJ, Goos M, et al. Transanal endoscopic tube decompression of acute colonic obstruction: Experience with 51 cases. Surg Endosc Other Interv Tech 2008;22(3):683–8.
46. Chudzinski AP, Thompson EV, Ayscue JM. Acute colonic pseudoobstruction. Clin Colon Rectal Surg 2015;28(2):112.
47. Johnson CD, Rice RP, Kelvin FM, et al. The radiologic evaluation of gross cecal distension: emphasis on cecal ileus. AJR Am J Roentgenol 1985;145(6):1211–7.
48. Vanek VW, Al-Salti M. Acute pseudo-obstruction of the colon (Ogilvie's syndrome). An analysis of 400 cases. Dis Colon Rectum 1986;29(3):203–10.
49. Delgado-Aros S, Camilleri M. Pseudo-obstruction in the critically ill. Bailliere's Best Pract Res Clin Gastroenterol 2003;17(3):427–44.
50. Stewart J, Finan PJ, Courtney DF, et al. Does a water soluble contrast enema assist in the management of acute large bowel obstruction: a prospective study of 117 cases. Br J Surg 1984;71(10):799–801.
51. Strodel WE, Nostrant TT, Dent TL. Therapeutic and diagnostic colonoscopy in nonobstructive colonic dilatation. Ann Surg 1983. https://doi.org/10.1097/00000 658-198304000-00007.
52. Rex DK. Colonoscopy and acute colonic pseudo-obstruction. Gastrointest Endosc Clin N Am 1997;7(3):499–508.
53. Geller A, Petersen BT, Gostout CJ. Endoscopic decompression for acute colonic pseudo-obstruction. Gastrointest Endosc 1996;44(2):144–50.
54. Harig JM, Fumo DE, Loo FD, et al. Treatment of acute nontoxic megacolon during colonoscopy: tube placement versus simple decompression. Gastrointest Endosc 1988;34(1):23–7.
55. Sgouros SN, Vlachogiannakos J, Vassiliadis K, et al. Effect of polyethylene glycol electrolyte balanced solution on patients with acute colonic pseudo obstruction after resolution of colonic dilation: a prospective, randomised, placebo controlled trial. Gut 2006;55(5):638–42.
56. Kahi CJ, Rex DK. Bowel obstruction and pseudo-obstruction. Gastroenterol Clin North Am 2003;32(4):1229–47.
57. VanSonnenberg E, Varney RR, Casola G, et al. Percutaneous cecostomy for Ogilvie syndrome: laboratory observations and clinical experience. Radiology 1990; 175(3):679–82.
58. Cowlam S, Watson C, Elltringham M, et al. Percutaneous endoscopic colostomy of the left side of the colon. Gastrointest Endosc 2007;65(7):1007–14.
59. Ramage JI, Baron TH. Percutaneous endoscopic cecostomy: A case series. Gastrointest Endosc 2003;57(6):752–5.
60. Bertolini D, De Saussure P, Chilcott M, et al. Severe delayed complication after percutaneous endoscopic colostomy for chronic intestinal pseudo-obstruction: A case report and review of the literature. World J Gastroenterol 2007;13(15): 2255.
61. Bray F, Ferlay J, Soerjomataram I, et al. Global cancer statistics 2018: GLOBOCAN estimates of incidence and mortality worldwide for 36 cancers in 185 countries. CA Cancer J Clin 2018;68(6):394–424.
62. Høydahl Ø, Edna TH, Xanthoulis A, et al. Long-term trends in colorectal cancer: incidence, localization, and presentation. BMC Cancer 2020;20(1):1–13.
63. Ansaloni L, Andersson RE, Bazzoli F, et al. Guidelenines in the management of obstructing cancer of the left colon: Consensus conference of the world society

of emergency surgery (WSES) and peritoneum and surgery (PnS) society. World J Emerg Surg 2010;5(1):1–10.

64. Decker KM, Lambert P, Nugent Z, et al. Time trends in the diagnosis of colorectal cancer with obstruction, perforation, and emergency admission after the introduction of population-based organized screening. JAMA Netw Open 2020;3(5): e205741.

65. Adler DG, Baron TH. Endoscopic palliation of colorectal cancer. Hematol Oncol Clin North Am 2002;16(4):1015–29.

66. Frago R, Ramirez E, Millan M, et al. Current management of acute malignant large bowel obstruction: a systematic review. Am J Surg 2014. https://doi.org/10.1016/j.amjsurg.2013.07.027.

67. Krukowskl ZH, Irwin ST. Malignant obstruction of the left colon. Br JournalofSutgety 1994;81:1270–6.

68. Yoo RN, Cho HM, Kye BH. Management of obstructive colon cancer: Current status, obstacles, and future directions. World J Gastrointest Oncol 2021;13(12): 1850.

69. Araki Y, Isomoto H, Matsumoto A, et al. Endoscopic decompression procedure in acute obstructing colorectal cancer. Endoscopy 2000;32(8):641–3.

70. Horiuchi A, Maeyama H, Ochi Y, et al. Usefulness of dennis colorectal tube in endoscopic decompression of acute, malignant colonic obstruction. Gastrointest Endosc 2001;54(2):229–32.

71. Jin SC, Sung WC, Kwang BP, et al. Interventional management of malignant colorectal obstruction: use of covered and uncovered stents. Korean J Radiol 2007; 8(1):57–63.

72. Van Hooft JE, Veld JV, Arnold D, et al. Self-expandable metal stents for obstructing colonic and extracolonic cancer: European Society of Gastrointestinal Endoscopy (ESGE) Guideline - Update 2020. Endoscopy 2020;52(5):389–407.

73. Watt AM, Faragher IG, Griffin TT, et al. Self-expanding metallic stents for relieving malignant colorectal obstruction: a systematic review. Ann Surg 2007;246(1): 24–30.

74. Zhang Y, Shi J, Shi B, et al. Self-expanding metallic stent as a bridge to surgery versus emergency surgery for obstructive colorectal cancer: a meta-analysis. Surg Endosc 2012;26(1):110–9.

75. Oh HH, Hong JY, Kim DH, et al. Differences in clinical outcomes according to the time interval between the bridge to surgery stenting and surgery for left-sided malignant colorectal obstruction. World J Surg Oncol 2022;20(1):1–9.

76. Saito S, Yoshida S, Isayama H, et al. A prospective multicenter study on self-expandable metallic stents as a bridge to surgery for malignant colorectal obstruction in Japan: efficacy and safety in 312 patients. Surg Endosc 2016; 30(9):3976–86.

77. Young CJ, De-Loyde KJ, Young JM, et al. Improving quality of life for people with incurable large-bowel obstruction: randomized control trial of colonic stent insertion. Dis Colon Rectum 2015;58(9):838–49.

78. Tal AO, Friedrich-Rust M, Bechstein WO, et al. Self-expandable metal stent for malignant colonic obstruction: outcome in proximal vs. left sided tumor localization. Z Gastroenterol 2013;51(6):551–7.

79. Finlayson A, Hulme-Moir M. Palliative colonic stenting: a safe alternative to surgery in stage IV colorectal cancer. ANZ J Surg 2016;86(10):773–7.

80. Siddiqui A, Cosgrove N, Yan LH, et al. Long-term outcomes of palliative colonic stenting versus emergency surgery for acute proximal malignant colonic obstruction: a multicenter trial. Endosc Int Open 2017;5(4):E232.

81. Keswani RN, Azar RR, Edmundowicz SA, et al. Stenting for malignant colonic obstruction: a comparison of efficacy and complications in colonic versus extracolonic malignancy. Gastrointest Endosc 2009;69:675–80.
82. Faraz S, Salem SB, Schattner M, et al. Predictors of clinical outcome of colonic stents in patients with malignant large-bowel obstruction because of extracolonic malignancy. Gastrointest Endosc 2018;87(5):1310–7.
83. Gevers AM, Macken E, Hiele M, et al. Endoscopic laser therapy for palliation of patients with distal colorectal carcinoma: analysis of factors influencing long-term outcome. Gastrointest Endosc 2000;51(5):580–5.
84. Solecki R, Zajac A, Richter P, et al. Bifocal esophageal and rectal cancer palliatively treated with argon plasma coagulation. Surg Endosc 2004;18(2):346.
85. Courtney ED, Raja A, Leicester RJ. Eight years experience of high-powered endoscopic diode laser therapy for palliation of colorectal carcinoma. Dis Colon Rectum 2005;48(4):845–50.

Endoscopic Management of Tumor Bleeding

Techniques and Strategies

Frances Dang, MD, MSc[a],*, Marc Monachese, MD, MSc[b]

KEYWORDS

- Tumor bleeding • Endoscopy • Hemostasis • Mechanical hemostasis
- Argon plasma coagulation • Topical hemostatic agents

KEY POINTS

- Tumor bleeding is a common and difficult challenge for the endoscopist despite improvements in technology and options for hemostasis.
- The evidence for optimal modality or technique for tumor bleeding remains limited. Guidelines do not support one modality over the other and the endoscopist must use all tools at their disposal.
- Electrotherapy (argon plasma coagulation [APC], cautery) has previously been the most effective option for the ability to treat a broad area. Newer topical hemostatic agents provide an additional option with good efficacy.
- Rebleeding rates and mortality remain high despite endoscopic therapy. Multidisciplinary discussions for management are crucial in these scenarios as surgical and/or radiologic interventions may be required.

INTRODUCTION

Gastrointestinal (GI) tumor bleeding can occur in the setting of primary GI tumors, locally invasive disease, or metastatic disease to the GI tract.[1] Bleeding due to GI tumor can vary in presentation, from occult bleeding to massive hemorrhage.[2] Traditionally, the role of endoscopic therapy for management of non-variceal GI bleeding has been shown to improve outcomes but this is less favorable in the context of tumor-related GI bleeding, which accounts for approximately 12% to 15% of all acute GI hemorrhage.[3,4,5] The effectiveness of conventional endoscopic therapy in tumor-related bleeding is variable and historically, obtaining durable control of tumor bleeding has been challenging due to limited options. The literature shows significant

a University of Toronto, 6 Queen's Park Crescent West, Third Floor, Toronto, Ontario, M5S 3H2, Canada; b Trillium Health Partners, 101 Queensway West, Unit 200, Mississauga, Ontario, L5B2P7, Canada
* Corresponding author.
E-mail address: fdang@qmed.ca

Gastrointest Endoscopy Clin N Am 34 (2024) 155–166
https://doi.org/10.1016/j.giec.2023.07.005
1052-5157/24/© 2023 Elsevier Inc. All rights reserved.

variance in the degree of success with hemostatic control, with initial hemostasis 80% to 100%, short-term rebleeding rate of 80%, and 30-day and 90-day mortality of 45% and 95%, respectively.[2,3,6,7]

Unfortunately, the data on endoscopic therapies for management of tumor bleeding are limited. Many of the earlier studies are single-center or multicenter retrospective reviews. Original device design and trials for hemostatic clips and electrotherapy tools were designed for non-malignant GI bleeding and their use has been adapted to tumor bleeding. There are very few dedicated randomized control trials with regards to evaluation of hemostasis of tumor bleeding but more recently, dedicated studies have been put forward specifically in evaluating hemostatic agents, which will be discussed later in this article. This provides an opportunity to re-evaluate the expected outcomes in managing these patients.

This article will explore all components of managing tumor bleeding broken down by modality, which are applicable to various tumors alongthe GI tract. The authors will highlight the advantages and disadvantages of each and how they may be applied. A review of available devices in the United States with video summaries on use and application can be seen at (Devices for endoscopic hemostasis of nonvariceal GI bleeding (with videos) - VideoGIE)[8]

INITIAL ASSESSMENT

When cancer patients present with upper GI bleed (UGIB), initial assessments should be performed according to general guidelines for the management of UGIB.[9,10] The initial assessment and pre-procedure planning are an important aspect in managing patients with active bleeding. The purpose of pre-procedure planning is to optimize the patient's condition and maximize the chance that endoscopic intervention is safe and effective. Planning includes a comprehensive evaluation of the patient's medical history, physical examination, laboratory tests, imaging studies, and any prior endoscopic findings. Imaging studies such as computed tomography (CT) and MRI can help determine the extent of the tumor and its relationship to adjacent structures. Laboratory tests including complete blood count (CBC), coagulation profile, and liver function tests can provide valuable information about a patient's overall health status, acuity of bleeding and if transfusion of blood products is required prior to endoscopic intervention. Similar to non-tumor bleeding, it is recommended that patients should receive blood and platelets to target a hemoglobin of 70 g/L and platelet count of 50,000, respectively.[9]

Risk stratifying patients for the need of urgent endoscopic therapy should be performed. Risk stratification tools such as the Rockall Score, AIMS65, and Glasgow Blatchford Score (GBS) have been well validated in non-tumor bleeding. A recent study evaluating these scores in the setting of GI tumor bleeding showed AIMS65 best predicted ICU admission and in-hospital mortality (AUC 0.85) in cases with upper GI cancers.[11] The GBS was most accurate in identifying the need for transfusion (AUC0.82) and low-risk group at admission (AUC 0.92). A new score was designed which was superior in predicting the need for hemostatic therapy (AUC 0.74) but further validation is required. All scores failed to predict hemostatic therapy and rebleeding.[11]

Once the source and extent of the bleeding have been determined, the next step is to develop a treatment plan. The choice of treatment depends on several factors, including the location and size of the tumor, the patient's overall health status, and the presence of comorbidities. It is currently unclear whether endoscopic therapy truly impacts outcomes with cancer-related bleeding. Given its lower invasiveness, endoscopic therapy is often the preferred initial treatment as it may avert the need for emergent surgery or temporize bleeding enough for patients to undergo further assessment for treatment.

OVERVIEW OF ENDOSCOPIC TECHNIQUES FOR TUMOR BLEEDING

Endoscopic techniques for controlling tumor bleeding include injection therapy, thermal therapy, mechanical therapy and more recently, hemostatic barriers (**Table 1**). Injection therapy involves the injection of substances such as epinephrine or sclerosants directly into the bleeding vessel to induce vasoconstriction or thrombosis. Thermal therapy includes the use of modalities such as laser, argon plasma coagulation (APC), and bipolar electrocoagulation to induce coagulation and tissue destruction. Mechanical therapy involves the use of clips, coils, or stents to mechanically occlude the bleeding vessel. Hemostatic barrier therapy involves applying a powder agent that on contact with blood polymerizes making a barrier to promote hemostasis.

INJECTION THERAPY

Injection therapy involves the injection of substances such as epinephrine, ethanol, or sclerosants directly into the bleeding vessel to induce vasoconstriction or thrombosis. Epinephrine is the most commonly used injection agent for tumor bleeding control. The use of injection of epinephrine was first described by Hirao and colleagues as prophylaxis of post-resection bleeding in gastric cancer.[12] It has later been used in the context of GI tumor bleeding given its proposed mechanism of action of local vasoconstriction, vascular tamponade, and thrombogenesis from edema and fibrinoid degeneration of the arterial wall.[10,13] The recommended concentration for epinephrine injection is 1:10,000, with higher volumes (>13 cc) shown to be effective in achieving hemostasis.[14] Injection of epinephrine is mostly used as adjunctive therapy as it has been shown that additional endoscopic treatment after epinephrine injection reduces further bleeding and the need for surgery in patients with high-risk bleeding peptic ulcers.[15] This concept is also generally applied to tumor bleeding as more endoscopic therapies have become available.

Injection of ethanol was first developed by Asaki on the premise of dehydration and fixation of tissue resulting in necrosis of the endothelial wall allowing for thrombogenesis.[16] Kim and colleagues describe a case of a patient who developed duodenal bleeding due to hepatocellular carcinoma (HCC) invasion, which was successfully treated with endoscopic injection of ethanol.[17] Overall, ethanol injection has fallen out of favor as monotherapy by more modern techniques given questions about efficacy and safety. Only small amounts are recommended as high concentrations have shown to increase the risk of perforation.[16]

Cyanoacrylates are a class of synthetic glues that solidify on contact with weak bases. There are case series describing the use of endoscopic ultrasound (EUS) to

Table 1			
Endoscopic modalities used for treatment of tumor bleeding in the gastrointestinal tract			
Injection	Mechanical	Thermal	Hemostatic Agents
Dilute epinephrine	Clips	Electrocautery	Hemospray
Ethanol	Endoloops	Argon plasma coagulation	Purastat
N-butyl-2-cyanoacrylate	Band Ligators	Radio frequency ablation	Nexpowder

directly inject cyanoacrylate (3–5 mL) into bleeding gastrointestinal stromal tumors (GIST).[18] Several other case series describe the use of topical sprayed cyanoacrylate glue via injection needle to achieve hemostasis in GI tumors (gastric, colon, and duodenal cancer) that were initially not controlled with epinephrine injection.[19–21] Generally, 1 ampule (0.5 mL) of histoacryl (n−butyl−2−cyanoacrylate) is used to achieve hemostasis. The histoacryl immediately forms white crystals when contacted with blood, creating a strong seal over the bleeding lesion.[20] Although the use of cyanoacrylate spray is not used as a standard modality for endoscopic treatment of GI bleeding, it has shown to be effective as a rescue therapy for lesions that were difficult to control using conventional methods with low rates of recurrent bleeding.[20,21]

MECHANICAL THERAPY

The physical characteristics of tumors in the GI tract often present as bulky, friable, and ulcerated masses, which invite attempts at various forms of mechanical therapy for tamponade that include clips, coils, or stents. The goal of using clips is for pure tamponade of possible underlying vessel. Endoscopic clips are manufactured from several companies and come in various sizes, can be rotatable and be opened and closed before deployment.[22] More recently, the Over-The-Scope Clip (OTSC; Ovesco, Tubingen, Germany) endoscopic clipping device was designed for tissue approximation of fistulas, perforations, and has been used in refractory non-variceal GI bleeding.[23] Although particularly good for treating refractory bleeding from large ulcers, there are cases of it being used in bleeding GI tumor in the stomach and ulcerative carcinoma of the pancreas.[24]

Endoloops are disposable snares that can be placed around the base of a tumor or on top of an ulcerated lesion that is protruded. Tightening of the endoloop around the stalk helps to provide mechanical tamponade.[25] Kashani and colleagues describe management of a periampullary tumor from metastatic hepatocellular carcinoma that was managed by 2 endoloops placed 1 month apart that resulted in stabilization of tumor bleeding and hemoglobin levels.[26] Brkic describes management of active bleeding from GI stromal tumor from an ulcerated crater in the gastric fundus. An endoloop was placed around the base of the tumor with the top of the ulcerated lesion protruded. With tightening of the endoloop, there was no clinical recurrence of bleeding detected.[27] Therefore, the use of endoloops to provide hemostasis in active tumor bleeding is possible; but as tumor size increases, it becomes more difficult to place the endoloop around the tumor and control bleeding from larger vessels.

The role of self-expandable metallic stents (SEMS) has evolved to include tumor-related bleeding in the upper GI tract. There are several case series and reports of bleeding from ulcerated esophageal tumors that could not be stopped with conventional endoscopic therapy but stopped with use of placing fully covered SEMS. One series of 4 patients describes bleeding from esophageal tumor that was stopped with the use of SEMS.[28] Only 1 of the 4 patients developed rebleeding with removal of SEMS but hemostasis was achieved with placement of second one. A pilot study by Han and colleagues looked at using SEMS for refractory hemorrhages caused by esophageal cancer. A total of 20 metal stents were placed in 17 patients with hemostasis rate of 88.2%. In addition, there are several case reports of using SEMS in malignant duodenal bleeding.[29–32] D'Souza and colleagues were one of the first to report a case of refractory bleeding from a malignant duodenal ulcer in a patient with HCC that was successfully treated with placement of fully covered SEMS.[29] The patient had 2 previous attempts at endoscopic therapy with clips, epinephrine injection, gold probe as well as embolization of gastroduodenal artery by interventional radiology without success.[29] For bleeding from the common bile duct, whether related to tumor or not, a covered SEMS should be considered first line as endoscopic therapy as clipping, injection, and thermal methods are generally ineffective.[33] Kawaguchi and colleagues describe a case of hemobilia that was treated with placement of a fully covered SEMS in a patient with HCC and biliary invasion.[34] Therefore, it appears that SEMS placement can be considered both safe and effective in the management of certain scenarios of recurrent or refractory bleeding of GI tumors.

Lastly, the use of coils has been mostly described in the treatment of bleeding gastric varices and there have only been case reports of using deploying coils to manage tumor bleeding. Romero-Castro and colleagues report 2 cases of EUS-guided combined coil deployment and further injection of cyanoacrylate glue to target feeding vessel of bleeding GISTs.[35]

THERMAL THERAPY

Thermal therapy involves the use of modalities that generate coagulation and tissue destruction of the bleeding vessel. A variety of contact and non-contact modalities exist including contact thermal devices such as heater probes, multipolar electrocautery probes, the mono-polar probe, and coagulation forceps. Non-contact thermal techniques include the use of APC and laser coagulation.

APC is a non-contact thermal therapy modality that uses ionized argon gas to deliver thermal energy to the tissue, leading to coagulation and tissue destruction. APC is a preferred method for the management of tumor-related gastrointestinal bleeding. Early data from MD Anderson Cancer Center over 3 consecutive years showed that immediate hemostasis was achieved in all 10 (100%) patients with primary or metastatic gastrointestinal cancer with bleeding.[36] Similar case series have shown efficacy of APC control of UGIB .[37]

Interestingly, other studies have shown despite high initial hemostasis, 30-day rebleeding and 30-day mortality were no different in a group of 53 patients with actively bleeding tumors.[38] More recent reviews from the MD Anderson group by Abu-Sbeih and colleagues have shown that in 313 patients only 22.7% received endoscopic treatment. Of this group, APC was the most utilized modality with hemostasis achieved in 57.7%. However, there was no decrease in recurrent bleeding or mortality.[39] It was noted that monotherapy with epinephrine injection and mechanical hemostasis with clips were not effective compared to APC.[33]

There are no large-powered randomized trials comparing APC to other modalities. Data regarding the optimal settings for APC therapy including mode of energy delivery, power, and gas flow rate have been reported in single-center series (**Table 2**).[3] Gas flow should be set at the lowest possible rate for desired tissue effect to reduce the risk of complications. Both forced and pulsed current delivery can be used. Forced mode delivers continuous delivery of energy, resulting in more rapid hemostasis. Pulsed mode sends intermittent bursts of energy to the tissue, resulting in a more superficial effect.

Contact thermal therapy has become less commonly used compared to non-contact therapy (ie, APC) given its limited field of application, reduced initial hemostasis, and higher rebleeding rates. As where APC can be applied across a diffusely oozing mass, contact modalities rely on the combination of heat and coaptive thermocoagulation to seal a blood vessel. Many tumors though do not have a single ulcerated and exposed vessel to treat. Reports of heater probes and bipolar electrocautery have shown moderate-excellent initial hemostasis (67%–100% initial response) but with high bleeding rates of 33% to 80%.[40] In addition, patients in these studies often required use of adjunctive interventions.

Table 2
Reported argon plasma coagulation settings for bleeding control of gastrointestinal tumors

APC Settings	Site of Lesion	Initial Hemostasis	Patients	Study
0–70W, 1.5–2.0 L/min (esophageal/gastric) 40–50W, 1.5 L/min (duodenal lesions)	Esophageal, Gastric & Duodenal	73%	25	Martins et al,[38] 2016
35 W, 1.0 L/min	Upper & Lower	100%	10	Thosani et al,[36] 2014
70 W, 2.0 L/min	Gastric	60%	3	Akhtar et al,[37] 2000

Table adapted from Ofosu et al.[3]

Radiofrequency ablation (RFA) has emerged as a cornerstone therapy in management of Barretts esophagus and more recently deployed for the use of treatment and palliation of biliary malignancies and cystic pancreatic neoplasms.[41] The use of RFA for tumor-related bleeding has not been well reported. A pilot study by Vavra and colleagues demonstrated the use of RFA as adjunct treatment and to provide hemostasis in 12 patients with rectal cancer. In 2 patients, RFA was used as monotherapy with hemostasis achieved.[42]

TOPICAL HEMOSTATIC AGENTS

Topical hemostatic agents (THA) are powder-based agents that can be applied directly to the bleeding site during endoscopy. The powder is composed of a blend of inorganic and organic components that adhere to the bleeding site, forming a barrier that promotes hemostasis. The application of these agents is quick, easy, and it does not require specialized training.[43] With regards to tumor bleeding, they are attractive as they can cover a wide area and can control diffuse oozing when a clear ulcer/vessel to intervene on is not seen.

Multiple agents have recently come to the market including hemostatic powder TC-325 (Hemospray; Cook Medical, Winston-Salem, NC, USA), adhesive hemostatic powder (UI-EWD; Nextbiomedical, Incheon, Republic of Korea), Endoclot polysaccharide hemostatic system (EndoClot Plus Inc, Santa Clara, Calif, USA), and Ankaferd Blood Stopper (Mefar Ilaç Sanayi AS, Istanbul, Turkey), summarized in **Table 3**.[44] Recent data show that rebleeding rates for non-tumor bleeding are lower and are similar to those with standard endoscopic therapy.[43]

In a meta-analysis examining 16 studies with 530 patients, primary hemostasis was achieved in 94.1% of the patients, the incidence of early rebleeding was 13.9%, and 11.4% for delayed rebleeding after the use of THAs.[45] This represents a significant improvement compared to the literature reported rebleeding rates of 28.3% to 80% from traditional therapeutic measures for hemostasis.[6,40,46] In one of the few direct comparison studies, Pittayanon and colleagues compared 14-day rebleeding between tumors treated with hemospray and those with traditional modalities. The 14-day rebleeding rate in the Hemospray group was 3 times lower than the control group but not statistically significant (10% vs 30%; $P = .60$). Thirty-day mortality rate was 3 times lower than that of in the conventional therapy group but not significant (10% vs 30%, $P = .7$).[47] A large nationwide Spanish study showed a 90.3% success of intraprocedural hemostasis with hemospray in 48 tumors, the majority of which were adenocarcinomas.[48]

Table 3
Available topical hemostatic agents

	TC-325 (Hemospray)	Endoclot	Ui-EWD (NexPowder)	Ankaferd Blood Stopper	CEGP-003
Material	Inert mineral powder	Starch-based absorbable modified polymers	Succinic anhydride (ε-poly- (L-lysine)) and oxidized dextran.	Five plant herbal extract	Hydroxyethylcellulose with epidermal growth factor
Mechanism	Absorbs water, forming a mechanical barrier over the bleeding site concentrating clotting factors.	Gel matrix leading to dehydration concerning clotting factors accelerating clotting cascade	Forms adhesive gel forming a mechanical barrier.	Formation of an encapsulated protein network	Forms adhesive gel to create mechanical barrier and promote wound healing
Air Source	CO_2	Room Air	CO_2	Not required	CO_2
Requires Active Bleeding	Yes	No	No	Yes	Yes
FDA Approved	Yes	Yes	Yes	No	No

Table adapted from Jiang et al.[44]

Each topical agent has a unique mechanism but all promote a favorable environment for a stable hemostatic clot to develop with formation of an additional barrier in some instances. The challenge of using this modality is the sensitivity of the catheter to occluding both during insertion through the scope working channel and once in the lumen. Unique adaptations to overcome this have been proposed such as using bone wax and a 3-way stopcock to improve patency and application (Link to video: Bone wax-tipped catheter and 3-way stopcock to optimize hemostatic powder deployment - VideoGIE).[49]

Newer agents such as UI-EWD (Nexpowder, Medtronic, Minneapolis, Minnesota) have a proprietary non-clogging catheter, which helps overcome catheter occlusion and use air instead of CO_2 to limit dispersion and improve visualization. Studies in UGIB report immediate hemostasis in 96.4% and 30-day rebleeding in only 3.7% of the patients.[50] A study by Shin and colleagues examining UI-EWD as monotherapy or rescue in 41 patients with malignant bleeding reported an immediate hemostasis rate of 97.5% and a rebleeding rate of 22.5% in 28 days.[51]

Other topical modalities include PuraStat (PuraStat, 3D-Matrix, Europe Ltd, France), a synthetic peptide agent that forms a transparent hydrogel at neutral pH. Once PuraStat is applied to a bleeding area, it will rapidly form a hydrogel barrier to produce hemostasis. Compared to other THA, the advantages of this modality include its transparent application allowing additional therapy and reduced risk of delivery catheter occlusion. There are no available data for its use in tumor bleeding. Studies in patients with UGIB showed successful hemostasis in greater than 80% of lesions with rebleeding occurring in ≤17% of the patients.[52]

SUMMARY

Endoscopic management of GI tumor-related bleeding is challenging due to high rebleeding rates, poor tissue response to endoscopic therapies, altered wound healing, and underlying coagulopathy. It is unclear whether endoscopic treatment shows overall improvement in outcomes of disease as bleeding from GI tumors generally does not respond as well to endoscopic treatment compared to benign etiologies of bleeding.[53] However, endoscopic treatment may help reduce transfusion requirements, avoid surgery, and provide a temporary bridge to oncologic therapy.[1,53] Traditionally, endoscopic hemostatic therapy has involved the use of thermal or mechanical therapy in conjunction with injection therapy. However, newer topical agents have entered the market. Cases that fail endoscopic intervention may require surgical or radiologic intervention.

VIDEO LINKS

Devices for endoscopic hemostasis of non-variceal GI bleeding- https://www.ncbi. nlm.nih.gov/pmc/articles/PMC661632.

Bone wax-tipped catheter and 3-way stopcock to optimize hemostatic powder deployment – VideoGIE- https://www.videogie.org/article/S2468-4481(21)00109-0.

Endoscopic hemostatic spray for uncontrolled bleeding after complicated endoscopic mucosal resection or endoscopic submucosal dissection: a report of 2 cases - https://www.videogie.org/article/S2468-4481(21)00108-9/.

CLINICS CARE POINTS

- Cancer patients presenting with upper GI bleeding should be assessed and managed to general guidelines for UGIB.

- Patients should be rescuscitated adequately and receive transfusion with hemoglobin target of 70 g/L and platelet count of 50,000.
- Endoscopic management of tumour bleeding can involve a variety of modalities from injection, thermal and mechanical therapy to newer topical hemostatic agents. Choice of modality will be dependent on local expertise and availability of resources.
- Despite endoscopic therapy, cancer patients with upper GI bleeding face high rebleeding and mortality rates. Multidisciplinary discussions for management of cases are important.

DISCLOSURE

The authors of this article have no financial disclosures to declare.

REFERENCES

1. Imbesi JJ, Kurtz RC. A multidisciplinary approach to gastrointestinal bleeding in cancer patients. J Support Oncol 2005;3(2):101–10. Available at: http://www.ncbi.nlm.nih.gov/pubmed/15796441.
2. Schatz RA, Rockey DC. Gastrointestinal Bleeding Due to Gastrointestinal Tract Malignancy: Natural History, Management, and Outcomes. Dig Dis Sci 2017; 62(2):491–501.
3. Ofosu A, Ramai D, Latson W, et al. Endoscopic management of bleeding gastrointestinal tumors. Ann Gastroenterol 2019;32(4):346–51.
4. Shivshanker K, Chu DZ, Stroehlein JR, et al. Gastrointestinal hemorrhage in the cancer patient. Gastrointest Endosc 1983;29(4):273–5.
5. Yarris JP, Warden CR. Gastrointestinal bleeding in the cancer patient. Emerg Med Clin North Am 2009;27(3):363–79.
6. Savides TJ, Jensen DM, Cohen J, et al. Severe upper gastrointestinal tumor bleeding: endoscopic findings, treatment, and outcome. Endoscopy 1996; 28(2):244–8.
7. Kim Y-I, Choi IJ. Endoscopic management of tumor bleeding from inoperable gastric cancer. Clin Endosc 2015;48(2):121–7.
8. ASGE technology committee, Parsi MA, Schulman AR, et al. Devices for endoscopic hemostasis of nonvariceal GI bleeding (with videos). VideoGIE an Off video J Am Soc Gastrointest Endosc 2019;4(7):285–99.
9. Barkun AN, Bardou M, Kuipers EJ, et al. International consensus recommendations on the management of patients with nonvariceal upper gastrointestinal bleeding. Ann Intern Med 2010;152(2):101–13.
10. Hwang JH, Fisher DA, Ben-Menachem T, et al. The role of endoscopy in the management of acute non-variceal upper GI bleeding. Gastrointest Endosc 2012; 75(6):1132–8.
11. Franco MC, Jang S, da Costa Martins B, et al. Risk Stratification in Cancer Patients with Acute Upper Gastrointestinal Bleeding: Comparison of Glasgow-Blatchford, Rockall and AIMS65, and Development of a New Scoring System. Clin Endosc 2022;55(2):240–7.
12. Hirao M, Masuda K, Asanuma T, et al. Endoscopic resection of early gastric cancer and other tumors with local injection of hypertonic saline-epinephrine. Gastrointest Endosc 1988;34(3):264–9.
13. Asge Technology Committee, Conway JD, Adler DG, et al. Endoscopic hemostatic devices. Gastrointest Endosc 2009;69(6):987–96.

14. Lin H-J, Hsieh Y-H, Tseng G-Y, et al. A prospective, randomized trial of large-versus small-volume endoscopic injection of epinephrine for peptic ulcer bleeding. Gastrointest Endosc 2002;55(6):615–9.
15. Vergara M, Bennett C, Calvet X, et al. Epinephrine injection versus epinephrine injection and a second endoscopic method in high-risk bleeding ulcers. Cochrane Database Syst Rev 2014;10:CD005584.
16. Asaki S, Nishimura T, Satoh A, et al. Endoscopic hemostasis of gastrointestinal hemorrhage by local application of absolute ethanol: a clinical study. Tohoku J Exp Med 1983;141(4):373–83.
17. Kim JN, Lee HS, Kim SY, et al. Endoscopic treatment of duodenal bleeding caused by direct hepatocellular carcinoma invasion with an ethanol injection. Gut Liver 2012;6(1):122–5.
18. Levy MJ, Wong K, Song LM, et al. Endoscopic ultrasound (EUS)-guided angiotherapy of refractory gastrointestinal bleeding. Am J Gastroenterol 2008;103(2): 352–9.
19. Prachayakul V, Aswakul P, Kachinthorn U. Spraying N-butyl-2-cyanoacrylate (Histoacryl) as a rescue therapy for gastrointestinal malignant tumor bleeding after failed conventional therapy. Endoscopy 2011;43(Suppl 2):E227–8.
20. Shida T, Takano S, Miyazaki M. Spraying n-butyl-2-cyanoacrylate (Histoacryl) might be a simple and final technique for bleeding gastrointestinal lesions. Endoscopy 2009;41(Suppl 2):E27–8.
21. Toapanta-Yanchapaxi L, Chavez-Tapia N, Téllez-Ávila F. Cyanoacrylate spray as treatment in difficult-to-manage gastrointestinal bleeding. World J Gastrointest Endosc 2014;6(9):448–52.
22. Romagnuolo J. Endoscopic clips: past, present and future. Can J Gastroenterol 2009;23(3):158–60.
23. Qiu J, Xu J, Zhang Y, et al. Over-the-Scope Clip Applications as First-Line Therapy in the Treatment of Upper Non-variceal Gastrointestinal Bleeding, Perforations, and Fistulas. Front Med 2022;9:753956.
24. Chan SM, Chiu PWY, Teoh AYB, et al. Use of the Over-The-Scope Clip for treatment of refractory upper gastrointestinal bleeding: a case series. Endoscopy 2014;46(5):428–31.
25. Arezzo A, Verra M, Miegge A, et al. Loop-and-let-go technique for a bleeding, large sessile gastric gastrointestinal stromal tumor (GIST). Endoscopy 2011; 43(Suppl 2):E18–9.
26. Kashani A, Nissen NN, Guindi M, et al. Metastatic Periampullary Tumor from Hepatocellular Carcinoma Presenting as Gastrointestinal Bleeding. Case Rep Gastrointest Med 2015;2015:732140.
27. Brkic T, Kalauz M, Ivekovic H. Endoscopic hemostasis using endoloop for bleeding gastric stromal tumor. Clin Gastroenterol Hepatol 2009;7(9):e53–4.
28. Zhou Y, Huo J, Wang X, et al. Covered -expanding metal stents for the treatment of refractory esophageal nonvariceal bleeding: a case series. J Laparoendosc Adv Surg Tech 2014;24(10):713–7.
29. D'Souza PM, Sandha GS, Teshima CW. Refractory bleeding from a malignant duodenal ulcer treated with placement of a fully-covered gastroduodenal stent. Dig Dis Sci 2013;58(11):3359–61.
30. Yen H-H, Chen Y-Y, Su P-Y. Successful use of a fully covered metal stent for refractory bleeding from a duodenal cancer. Endoscopy 2015;47(Suppl 1):E34–5.
31. Orii T, Karasawa Y, Kitahara H, et al. Efficacy of Self-Expandable Metallic Stent Inserted for Refractory Hemorrhage of Duodenal Cancer. Case Rep Gastroenterol 2016;10(1):151–6.

32. Daiku K, Ikezawa K, Maeda S, et al. A case of refractory tumor bleeding from an ampullary adenocarcinoma: Compression hemostasis with a self-expandable metallic stent. DEN open 2022;2(1):e23.
33. Sugimoto M, Takagi T, Suzuki R, et al. The Dramatic Haemostatic Effect of Covered Self-expandable Metallic Stents for Duodenal and Biliary Bleeding. Intern Med 2021;60(6):883–9.
34. Kawaguchi Y, Ogawa M, Maruno A, et al. A case of successful placement of a fully covered metallic stent for hemobilia secondary to hepatocellular carcinoma with bile duct invasion. Case Rep Oncol 2012;5(3):682–6.
35. Romero-Castro R, Jimenez-Garcia VA, Irisawa A, et al. Endoscopic ultrasound-guided angiotherapy in bleeding gastrointestinal stromal tumors with coil deployment and cyanoacrylate injection. Endoscopy 2021;53(4):E124–5.
36. Thosani N, Rao B, Ghouri Y, et al. Role of argon plasma coagulation in management of bleeding GI tumors: evaluating outcomes and survival. Turk J Gastroenterol 2014;25(Suppl 1):38–42.
37. Akhtar K, Byrne JP, Bancewicz J, et al. Argon beam plasma coagulation in the management of cancers of the esophagus and stomach. Surg Endosc 2000; 14(12):1127–30.
38. Martins BC, Wodak S, Gusmon CC, et al. Argon plasma coagulation for the endoscopic treatment of gastrointestinal tumor bleeding: A retrospective comparison with a non-treated historical cohort. United Eur Gastroenterol J 2016;4(1):49–54.
39. Abu-Sbeih H, Szafron D, Elkafrawy AA, et al. Endoscopy for the diagnosis and treatment of gastrointestinal bleeding caused by malignancy. J Gastroenterol Hepatol 2022;37(10):1983–90.
40. Loftus EV, Alexander GL, Ahlquist DA, et al. Endoscopic treatment of major bleeding from advanced gastroduodenal malignant lesions. Mayo Clin Proc 1994;69(8):736–40.
41. Gollapudi LA, Tyberg A. EUS-RFA of the pancreas: where are we and future directions. Transl Gastroenterol Hepatol 2022;7:18.
42. Vavra P, Dostalik J, Zacharoulis D, et al. Endoscopic radiofrequency ablation in colorectal cancer: initial clinical results of a new bipolar radiofrequency ablation device. Dis Colon Rectum 2009;52(2):355–8.
43. Chen Y-I, Barkun AN. Hemostatic Powders in Gastrointestinal Bleeding: A Systematic Review. Gastrointest Endosc Clin N Am 2015;25(3):535–52.
44. Jiang SX, Chahal D, Ali-Mohamad N, Kastrup C, Donnellan F. Hemostatic powders for gastrointestinal bleeding: a review of old, new, and emerging agents in a rapidly advancing field. Endosc Int open 2022;10(8):E1136–46. https://doi.org/10.1055/a-1836-8962.
45. Karna R, Deliwala S, Ramgopal B, et al. Efficacy of topical hemostatic agents in malignancy-related GI bleeding: a systematic review and meta-analysis. Gastrointest Endosc 2023;97(2):202–8.e8.
46. Song IJ, Kim HJ, Lee JA, et al. Clinical Outcomes of Endoscopic Hemostasis for Bleeding in Patients with Unresectable Advanced Gastric Cancer. J Gastric Cancer 2017;17(4):374–83.
47. Pittayanon R, Prueksapanich P, Rerknimitr R. The efficacy of Hemospray in patients with upper gastrointestinal bleeding from tumor. Endosc Int Open 2016; 4(9):E933–6.
48. Rodríguez de Santiago E, Burgos-Santamaría D, Pérez-Carazo L, et al. Hemostatic spray powder TC-325 for GI bleeding in a nationwide study: survival and predictors of failure via competing risks analysis. Gastrointest Endosc 2019; 90(4):581–90.e6.

49. Tau JA, Imam Z, Bazerbachi F. Bone wax-tipped catheter and 3-way stopcock to optimize hemostatic powder deployment. VideoGIE an Off video J Am Soc Gastrointest Endosc 2021;6(9):387–9.
50. Park J-S, Kim HK, Shin YW, et al. Novel hemostatic adhesive powder for nonvariceal upper gastrointestinal bleeding. Endosc Int Open 2019;7(12):E1763–7.
51. Shin J, Cha B, Park J-S, et al. Efficacy of a novel hemostatic adhesive powder in patients with upper gastrointestinal tumor bleeding. BMC Gastroenterol 2021; 21(1):40.
52. Branchi F, Klingenberg-Noftz R, Friedrich K, et al. PuraStat in gastrointestinal bleeding: results of a prospective multicentre observational pilot study. Surg Endosc 2022;36(5):2954–61.
53. Heller SJ, Tokar JL, Nguyen MT, et al. Management of bleeding GI tumors. Gastrointest Endosc 2010;72(4):817–24.

Endoscopic Nutrition of Patients with Cancer

Kinnari Modi, MD[a], David Lee, MD, MPH[b],*

KEYWORDS

- Nasogastric tube • Enteral stents • Percutaneous endoscopic gastrostomy tubes
- Endoscopic ultrasound-guided gastroenterostomy

KEY POINTS

- A wide range of endoscopic therapies are available to aid in maintaining nutritional status in patients with cancer.
- Endoscopic placement of a nasogastric tube or nasoenteral tube can be a simple solution for those patients in whom the length of oral intake impairment is expected to be short, typically less than 30 days.
- Percutaneous endoscopic gastrostomy tubes are durable, longer term solutions for patients requiring nutritional support with intact, functional gastrointestinal tracts.
- Self-expanding metal stents have been successfully used to restore patency of the esophagus, duodenum, and colon, typically for palliative relief of obstructive symptoms in advanced incurable malignancy.
- There is a growing body of literature showing excellent results with endoscopic ultrasound-guided gastroenterostomies as a means of relieving gastric outlet obstruction.

INTRODUCTION

Maintaining a patient's nutritional status is a fundamental objective throughout the course of cancer treatment. And yet, malignancy-associated cachexia remains a common problem encountered in patients with cancer. It is associated with poorer response to therapy, worsened quality of life, and poor short-term and long-term outcomes.[1] Therefore, it has been of critical importance to encourage patients to maintain their oral intake throughout the treatment process and supplement their intake when necessary in order to maintain their nutritional status.

Despite these measures, many patients with cancer will be unable to maintain adequate oral intake on their own, requiring additional means for providing nutrition. This may be due to general debility and deconditioning related to the cancer and its

a Department of Internal Medicine, Methodist Dallas Medical Center, Dallas, TX, USA;
b Methodist Digestive Institute, Methodist Dallas Medical Center, Dallas, TX, USA
* Corresponding author. 221 West Colorado Boulevard, Pavilion II, Suite 630, Dallas, TX 75208.
E-mail address: davidlee@mhd.com

Gastrointest Endoscopy Clin N Am 34 (2024) 167–177
https://doi.org/10.1016/j.giec.2023.09.010
1052-5157/24/© 2023 Elsevier Inc. All rights reserved.

treatment or more directly due to obstruction of part of the alimentary tract from the malignancy itself.

There have been a variety of endoscopic interventions that have been developed to maintain enteral access for continued nutrition. In this review, the authors discuss the various endoscopic interventions available for maintaining nutrition in patients with cancer.

DISCUSSION
Endoscopic Nasogastric Tube Placement

The nasogastric tube (NGT)/nasoenteral tube (NET) is a commonly used appliance to achieve enteral access in patients. The provision of nutrition via NGT/NET is most appropriate for patients in whom the length of impaired oral intake is expected to be short, typically estimated at less than 30 days.

Typically, these are placed at bedside without the need for endoscopic assistance. However, inability to place NGT/NET due to difficult anatomy or an obstruction along the path of the tube could necessitate placement under endoscopic visualization.

A variety of techniques have been described to aid in endoscopic placement of these tubes. The simplest involves passage of a gastroscope to the level of the obstruction and subsequent passage of the NGT/NET through the residual lumen of the obstruction under direct endoscopic visualization.

In cases where the anatomy impedes the placement of the tube, a variety of adjunctive techniques have been described.[2] In the "drag and pull" technique, a suture is secured to the tip of the NET, which is grasped by an instrument passed through the working channel of the endoscope. The tube is then passed with the endoscope into position. In the "over the guidewire" technique, a guidewire is passed through the endoscope and then exchanged out. The NET is then passed over the guidewire into position. Finally, the use of an ultraslim gastroscope passed transnasally has been described to allow for through-the-scope placement of a NET.[3] This has been noted to be especially helpful for patients with high-grade obstruction related to esophageal cancer, reporting a 99% success rate and no complications.

Overall, the endoscopic placement of NGT/NET remains a fundamental option for establishing enteral access in patients with cancer. With more modern technological advancements, though, the need for endoscopy is being supplanted by bedside techniques. For example, the development of weighted NETs with an electromagnetic tip allows for real-time imaging of the placement of the NET via sensors attached to the lower chest wall and has become commonplace in many facilities.[4]

Percutaneous Endoscopic Gastrostomy Tube Placement

Percutaneous endoscopic gastrostomy (PEG) tube placement has become a preferred means of establishing long-term enteral access in patients who are unable to meet their nutritional needs per-orally.

There are three main techniques for PEG tube placement: the Gauderer-Ponsky pull method, the Sachs-Vine push method, and the Russell introducer method. Among these, the Gauderer-Ponsky and the Sachs-Vine methods are the most commonly used.

In the Gauderer-Ponsky pull method, first described in 1980,[5] the gastroscope is first advanced to the stomach, and the stomach is fully insufflated to oppose the anterior stomach with the abdominal wall. After locating an appropriate site for placement via transillumination and/or manual pressure, a trocar needle is placed percutaneously into the gastric lumen. A guidewire is then passed through the trocar and ensnared by the gastroscope. The endoscope along with the ensnared guidewire is then pulled out of the mouth. The PEG tube is then attached to the guidewire via a loop of suture, and the guidewire is slowly pulled out of the abdominal wall, thus pulling the PEG tube down through the patient's mouth and down into the stomach before emerging from the anterior abdominal wall.

The Sachs-Vine push method is similar to the Gauderer-Ponsky pull method except that the PEG tube is a semirigid, tapered tube with a dilator at the end. The dilator is passed over the guidewire and pushed out through the abdominal wall at the incision site.

In the Russell introducer method,[6,7] the stomach is insufflated, and a needle is placed through the abdominal wall into the stomach, similar to the previous methods. A J-shaped guidewire is passed through the needle, and an introducer sheath and dilator are pushed over the guidewire. The sheath remains in place, and the guidewire and dilator are removed. A balloon-tipped PEG tube is then placed through the introducer sheath; the catheter balloon is inflated and pulled against the abdominal wall bringing the stomach wall into position with the abdominal wall.

PEG tubes have been associated with improved outcomes, especially in those individuals with poorer nutritional status at the start of treatment. A recent study involved a large, multicenter retrospective analysis of 904 patients[8] with head and neck cancers who received prophylactic PEG tube placement versus no PEG tube. The study compared weight loss and treatment tolerance between these two groups, and found overall, the differences between the two groups were nonsignificant for weight loss and treatment tolerance. However, a subgroup of patients with PEG tube placement who had BMI less than 18.5 kg/m^2 undergoing non-intensity-modulated radiation therapy were able to tolerate the therapy better than the non-PEG tube placement.

In another prospective study, 133 patients with noninvasive metastatic nasopharyngeal cancer who were treated with prophylactic PEG tube placement were found to have significant improvement in terms of completion of chemotherapy, less weight loss, and lower incidence of mucositis than those in the non-PEG tube group.[9]

An alternate role for PEG tube in malignancy is for gastric decompression in cases of malignant gastric outlet obstruction. Malignant gastric outlet obstruction can cause significant nausea and vomiting in patients with end-stage cancer. In such patients, PEG tube placement can be considered for decompression. Multiple smaller studies have been conducted to study the symptomatic outcomes for PEG tube placement for decompression in patients with cancer. In one small study, six out of seven patients had instant relief of nausea and vomiting the first day after PEG placement.[10] One of the patients developed cellulitis and needed to have their PEG tube removed at 11 months. The mean survival in these six patients after PEG tube placement was 119 days.

In a larger prospective study,[11] 76 patients with malignant bowel obstruction underwent PEG tube placement for decompression of which 69% had successful PEG tube placement; 19% of patients had complications including PEG tube site leakage and wound infection.

A special note should be made of the risk of cancer seeding in PEG tube placement. Especially in cases of head/neck cancer or esophageal cancer, there is the risk of seeding of the cancer into the peritoneal cavity and metastasis due to the PEG tube being swept through the malignancy during the process of placement. The range of estimates for the risk of seeding is low, varying from less than 1% up to 9% in some studies.[12,13] A recent retrospective review[14] concluded that the risk of cancer seeding with PEG tube placement may be underestimated. The location of the tumor (eg, pharyngoesophageal), poorly differentiated tumor and large cancer sizes are risk factors for stomal metastasis of the tumor.

Overall, PEG tube placement is a safe and widely available procedure for long-term enteral access in patients with cancer. PEG tube placement can be used both for nutritional feeding in cases where oral intake is compromised and for palliative decompression in cases of end stage malignant gastric outlet obstruction. Given that there are both immediate risks associated with the procedure itself and long-term risks including the risk of cancer seeding, the decision to proceed with PEG tube placement should follow a thorough discussion of the risks versus benefits of this procedure with the patient.

Percutaneous Endoscopic Gastrostomy with Jejunal Extension and Percutaneous Endoscopic Jejunostomy Tube Placement

There are specific instances, where it may be preferable for enteral nutrition to be fed into the small bowel rather than gastric lumen. Generally, these would be instances of gastric outlet obstruction, the presence of gastroparesis, or surgically altered anatomy making gastric placement infeasible.

The PEG with jejunal extension (PEG-J) involves the use of a jejunal extension tube that is passed coaxially through the lumen of a PEG tube and subsequently maneuvered such that the tip is in the small bowel. The PEG-J has the advantage of providing access to both the gastric lumen and small bowel lumen, such that the gastric port can be used for decompression, whereas the jejunal port is used for feeding. However, the rather small caliber of the jejunal extension does mean the tube can be more prone to clogging.[15] In addition, the main drawback to the PEG-J has been the tendency for the jejunal extension to recoil back into the gastric lumen, thus negating the advantages of small bowel feeding. Various modifications have been made to the jejunal extension to try to minimize the risk of this recoiling effect, including the use of suture to allow for the distal tip to be clipped to the wall of the small bowel or the distal tip having a pigtail to help maintain position (**Fig. 1**). One interesting modification uses a pediatric PEG tube in place of the jejunal extension, with the internal bumper of the pediatric PEG tube acting as a sail to maintain position in the small bowel.[16]

An alternative to this method of jejunal access is the direct percutaneous endoscopic jejunostomy (PEJ) tube. This modifies the technique of PEG tube placement to percutaneously access a loop of small bowel, through which the feeding tube is placed.[17,18] The most technically challenging aspect of this technique is finding an appropriate loop of bowel that comes in close association to the anterior abdominal wall and then being able to accurately penetrate into this relatively small caliber lumen. This technique has, therefore, been described as more successful in those patients with lower body mass index (BMI) (less than 25), with higher BMI associated with lower rates of success and a higher rate of complications.[19]

A recent meta-analysis[20] comparing PEG-J with direct PEJ demonstrated that direct PEJ tubes have lower rates of tube malfunction and failure rates. However, they are technically more challenging to place and seem to have a greater learning curve compared with PEG-J. PEG-J is associated with higher rates of technical success at initial placement with native anatomy.

Currently, guidelines from both the American Society for Gastrointestinal Endoscopy and the European Society of Gastrointestinal Endoscopy support the use of PEJ and PEG-J tubes for long-term post-pyloric feeding as alternatives to nasojejunal tubes or surgical jejunostomies.[21,22] The decision to place these tubes will depend on the specific condition of the patient, including their anatomy and body habitus and the technical expertise of the endoscopist and resources available.

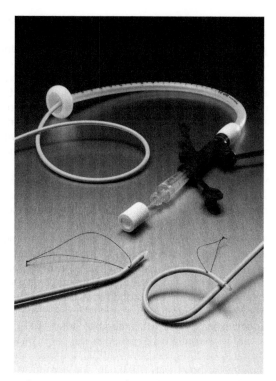

Fig. 1. Ex vivo image of a percutaneous endoscopic gastrostomy tube with jejunal extension (PEG-J). In the foreground are two different distal tips of the jejunal extension, both with built-in suture to clip to the jejunal wall. The version on the right has a pigtailed distal tip. These are to help prevent the jejunal extension from recoiling back into the stomach. (Image provided courtesy of Boston Scientific. ©2023 Boston Scientific Corporation or its affiliates. All rights reserved.)

Endoscopic Enteral Stenting

Endoscopic stent placement in patients with cancer is used to relieve symptomatic obstruction of the gastrointestinal (GI) tract. These stents have been used to maintain luminal patency in the esophagus, the duodenum, and the colon.

Esophageal stenting

Esophageal cancer is oftentimes associated with dysphagia. Indeed, it is not uncommon for dysphagia to be the first presenting symptom of esophageal cancer. Esophageal stenting is indicated for palliation of dysphagia and improvement in quality of life in patients who are not surgical candidates or with recurrent disease after primary treatment. The idea of placing a stent to relieve obstruction has been around since at least the late nineteenth century, with rigid stents having been made of various materials (wood, plastic, metal, and latex) over the years.[23] Modern esophageal stents are self-expanding metal stents (SEMSs) made of nitinol, an alloy of nickel and titanium. There is a wide range of esophageal stent models of various manufacturers, but these can generally be classified into one of three categories: uncovered metal stents, covered metal stents, and partially covered metal stents. Covered metal stents have the advantage of resisting tumor ingrowth and can be removed, such as in cases where the patient does not tolerate the stent. Uncovered metal stents have lower rates of migration in comparison to covered metal stents but can become occluded due to tumor ingrowth.[24] Partially covered stents usually have the body of the stent covered to resist tumor ingrowth while having exposed flanges that allow for this portion to embed into the mucosa to resist migration.

These stents come in a variety of lengths and diameters, which can be sized according to the dimensions of the obstruction. Generally, it is important to not traverse or come into close proximity of the upper esophageal sphincter due to the potential for impairing swallowing function and the potential for intolerable foreign body sensation. Traversing the lower esophageal sphincter (LES) should also be avoided unless it is absolutely necessary due to the severe reflux that ensues from stenting across the LES.

Endoscopic placement of these esophageal stents is generally performed under fluoroscopic guidance, after which these stents are allowed to fully expand over the next 24 to 48 hours of placement. Complications including chest pain, stent migration, bleeding, pneumonia, obstruction, and esophageal rupture can occur in about a third to half of patients, with estimates in studies ranging from 10.5% to 64.4%.[25]

Since the advent of modern esophageal SEMS, it has become widely used for the palliation of obstructive symptoms in esophageal malignancy. It has favorable outcomes for the improvement of dysphagia in comparison to photodynamic therapy, laser therapy, esophageal bypass, and rigid plastic stents. However, in comparison to PEG tube placement, there are some indications that SEMS placement may be inferior to PEG tubes for improving nutritional status and possibly overall survival. For example, in a retrospective study of 308 patients who underwent PEG tube placement versus SEMS placement for palliation in esophageal cancer,[26] those in the PEG tube group were found to have better survival ($P = .007$) and less need for intervention ($P < .001$) in comparison to those with SEMS. In another study of 113 patients,[27] PEG tube patients had a longer overall survival time compared with the SEMS group in stage II, III (201 vs 185 days, $P = .034$), and stage IV (122 vs 86 days, $P = .001$) esophageal cancer. The PEG tube placement group also had lower local post-procedure pain as well as lower incidence of dislodgement (1.5% vs 19.1%, $P = .002$). In both of these studies, patients in the PEG tube group also had higher albumin levels, a marker of nutritional status. Therefore, although PEG tubes do not palliate dysphagia symptoms, it may be a favorable alternative in comparison to SEMS placement in terms of maintaining nutrition and avoiding post-procedure complications and patients should be thoroughly counseled before proceeding with either course of action.

Duodenal stenting

Similar to esophageal stents, SEMSs have been used in the palliation of gastric outlet obstruction due to distal gastric tumors or duodenal obstruction, such as from pancreatic cancer, ampullary malignancy, or metastases. The goal in duodenal stenting is to relieve symptoms of gastric outlet obstruction, allow patients to resume oral intake, and improve quality of life.

In the United States, the SEMSs used in the duodenum are uncovered. Covered metal stents for the duodenum are available internationally. Uncovered metal stents have lower rates of migration in comparison to covered metal stents[28] and have the added advantage of allowing for biliary drainage through the open sidewall of the stent.

Particular nuances of duodenal stenting include the role of biliary drainage before duodenal stenting. It is not uncommon for tumors affecting gastric outlet to also cause biliary obstruction, such as tumors of the head/uncinate process of the pancreas. If there is evidence of jaundice or even impending biliary obstruction on imaging, it is reasonable to first place a biliary stent ahead of deploying a duodenal stent due to the difficulty of accessing the ampulla once a duodenal stent has been deployed over this area.[29]

Current guidelines suggest duodenal stenting for patients with a life expectancy of less than 6 months who desire resumption of oral intake with shorter length of stay in the hospital.[30] This is because while duodenal stents have been shown to have high rates of technical success for initial deployment, their long-term durability and efficacy seem to be inferior to surgical gastrojejunostomy (SGJ).[30–32]

Colonic stenting

Another location in which SEMS technology has been applied is for the palliation of obstruction related to colorectal malignancy. Colonic stenting is indicated for patients with advanced incurable malignancy for the palliation of colonic obstruction symptoms or for the decompression of the colon as a bridge to surgery. In the United States, only uncovered metal stents are available for colonic stenting, although covered stents are available internationally.

The placement of colonic stents has been shown to be an effective means for restoring patency to the colonic lumen. Care should be taken to avoid placing the colonic stent too low within the rectum due to the potential for causing severe rectal pain and tenesmus symptoms, though there have been some reports describing success in placing low-lying colonic stents with tolerable side effects.[33]

Overall, the risk of complications with colonic stenting is about 25% and includes the risks of stent migration, recurrent obstruction, and perforation. Among these, perforation is the most significant side effect and seems to occur when the stent is deployed in the sigmoid colon, where the radial forces from the stent within an angulated redundant colonic lumen increase the risk of focal pressure ischemia on the colonic wall.[34,35] Ongoing treatment of colorectal cancer may also increase this risk of perforation, and the use of the antiangiogenic agent bevacizumab in particular has been associated with higher rates of colonic perforation after stenting.[35] It has therefore been recommended to avoid colonic stenting in patients undergoing treatment with bevacizumab and related agents.[36]

Endoscopic Ultrasound-Guided Gastroenterostomy

The latest development in endoscopic techniques for maintaining enteral access is the endoscopic ultrasound-guided gastroenterostomy (EUS-GE).

The ability to perform a EUS-guided GE was proposed as far back as 2002[37] though in an animal model. The techniques and instruments available at the time were too cumbersome for clinical practice.

However, with the development of electrocautery-tipped lumen-apposing metal stents (LAMSs) (**Fig. 2**), the ability to safely bring together two luminal structures

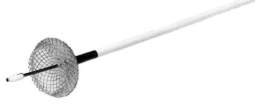

Fig. 2. Partially deployed electrocautery-tipped lumen apposing metal stent (Hot AXIOS stent). (Image provided courtesy of Boston Scientific. ©2023 Boston Scientific Corporation or its affiliates. All rights reserved.)

has been greatly expanded. Initially described for EUS-guided cystogastrostomy, there is an expanding body of literature describing the use of this device for a wide range of indications, from biliary and gallbladder drainage to gastroenterostomies.

First described by Binmoeller and Shah in an animal model,[38] the EUS-GE is an alternative to surgical bypass for palliation of malignant gastric outlet obstruction. The technique hinges on the ability to identify an appropriate loop of either distal duodenum or proximal jejunum from the gastric mucosa. Typically, an endoscopy is first performed ahead of the procedure in order to place a guidewire through the malignant obstruction, over which a water-instilling device is passed to the level of the anastomosis location. The loop of intestine is then instilled with water or saline, sometimes colored with methylene blue. Under endoscopic ultrasound visualization, the distended loop of bowel is then identified. When EUS-GE is performed with a guidewire, a 19-gauge needle is then used to puncture the stomach and the enteral loop, followed by a guidewire which is passed through the needle into the enteral lumen. The needle is then exchanged out for an electrocautery-tipped LAMS, which is deployed connecting the lumen of the stomach and the enteral loop.[39] More recent iterations of the technique have eliminated the need for the guidewire exchange in favor of a direct puncture using the electrocautery tip to deploy the LAMS directly.

This technique has provided excellent palliation of the symptoms of malignant gastric outlet obstruction in multiple studies. For example, there is a recent multicenter international study including 93 patients comparing clinical success, technical success, and adverse outcomes from EUS-GE versus SGJ.[40] Although the technical success rate was significantly higher in the SGJ group ($P < .009$), there was no difference in clinical success rate. The length of hospital stay was the same in both groups, and the EUS-GE group had a tendency toward less adverse events, although this was not statistically significant. Itoi and colleagues conducted a prospective study for 20 patients with malignancy outlet obstruction who underwent assisted EUS-GE with a technical success rate of 90%.[41]

A recent retrospective study compared EUS-GE with endoscopic stent placement in 103 patients with both benign and malignant gastric outlet obstruction.[42] There was no difference in the technical and clinical success and adverse events ($P = .4$) between both groups, but the EUS-GE group had a significantly lower need for unplanned re-intervention (HR: 0.264; 95% CI: 0.086, 0.813; $P = .02$).

Another retrospective multicenter study compared EUS-GE with SGJ for malignant gastric outlet obstruction.[43] This study included a total of 310 patients, with similar rates of technical success (97.9 vs 100%) and clinical success (94.1% vs 94.3%) but with higher re-intervention rates in the EUS-GE group (15.5% vs 1.63%, $P < .001$). People who underwent EUS-GE, however, had significantly sooner resumption of chemotherapy (16.6 days vs 37.8 days, $P < .001$) and sooner resumption of oral intake (1.4 vs 4.06 days, $P < .001$). In addition, the adverse event rate was lower for EUS-GE (13.4% vs 33.3%, $P < .001$).

Overall, EUS-GE is a novel and promising technique for the palliation of malignant gastric outlet obstruction. However, it is a technically challenging procedure that should be reserved for expert interventional endoscopists at centers with the expertise to handle such complex patients.

SUMMARY

In this review, the authors have sought to provide an overview of the multiple endoscopic interventions routinely used for maintaining nutritional needs in patients with cancer. The general principle for these interventions is to bypass the affected areas of the alimentary tract and make use of the unaffected areas of the alimentary tract to the greatest extent possible. The possible endoscopic solutions have expanded over the years, corresponding to advancements, and new developments in technology and technique and further evolution of available therapies are inevitably on the horizon.

CLINICS CARE POINTS

- Endoscopic placement of a nasogastric tube or nasoenteral tube can be a simple solution for patients in whom the length of oral intake impairment is expected to be short, typically less than 30 days. Longer duration of impairment should prompt consideration of alternative means of maintaining enteral access.

- Percutaneous endoscopic gastrostomy tubes provide durable longer term solutions for nutritional support. If there is impaired gastric emptying, a PEG-J can be considered, with a possible direct PEJ considered later if the patient tolerates jejunal feeding, and if the expertise of the endoscopist allows for this.

- Self-expanding metal stents have been successfully used to restore patency of the esophagus, duodenum, and colon in cases of malignant obstruction. Typically, these stents are meant for palliative relief of obstructive symptoms in advanced, incurable disease. Caution should be taken in patients undergoing active treatment with certain chemotherapy/radiation therapy regimens, especially in the colon.

- Endoscopic ultrasound-guided gastroenterostomies are showing great results as a means of relieving gastric outlet obstruction, but this is a technically challenging procedure that should be reserved for expert interventional endoscopists at higher levels centers.

DISCLOSURE

No disclosures.

REFERENCES

1. Arends J, Bachmann P, Baracos V, et al. ESPEN guidelines on nutrition in cancer patients. Clin Nutr 2017;36:11–48.
2. Rafferty GP, Tham TC. Endoscopic placement of enteral feeding tubes. World J Gastrointest Endosc 2010;2:155–64.
3. Lin CH, Liu NJ, Lee CS, et al. Nasogastric feeding tube placement in patients with esophageal cancer: application of ultrathin transnasal endoscopy. Gastrointest Endosc 2006;64:104–7.
4. Ackerman MH, Mick DJ. Technologic approaches to determining proper placement of enteral feeding tubes. AACN Adv Crit Care 2006;17:246–9.
5. Gauderer MW, Ponsky JL, Izant RJ Jr. Gastrostomy without laparotomy: a percutaneous endoscopic technique. J Pediatr Surg 1980;15:872–5.
6. Miller RE, Winkler WP, Kotler DP. The Russell percutaneous endoscopic gastrostomy: key technical steps. Gastrointest Endosc 1988;34:339–42.
7. Russell TR, Brotman M, Norris F. Percutaneous gastrostomy. A new simplified and cost-effective technique. Am J Surg 1984;148:132–7.
8. Dechaphunkul T, Ngamphaiboon N, Danchaivijitr P, et al. Benefits of prophylactic percutaneous gastrostomy in patients with nasopharyngeal cancer receiving concurrent chemoradiotherapy: A multicenter analysis. Am J Otolaryngol 2022;43:103356.
9. Xu Y, Guo Q, Lin J, et al. Benefit of percutaneous endoscopic gastrostomy in patients undergoing definitive chemoradiotherapy for locally advanced nasopharyngeal carcinoma. OncoTargets Ther 2016;9:6835–41.

10. Teriaky A, Gregor J, Chande N. Percutaneous endoscopic gastrostomy tube placement for end-stage palliation of malignant gastrointestinal obstructions. Saudi J Gastroenterol 2012;18:95–8.

11. Kawata N, Kakushima N, Tanaka M, et al. Percutaneous endoscopic gastrostomy for decompression of malignant bowel obstruction. Dig Endosc 2014;26:208–13.

12. Cappell MS. Risk factors and risk reduction of malignant seeding of the percutaneous endoscopic gastrostomy track from pharyngoesophageal malignancy: a review of all 44 known reported cases. Am J Gastroenterol 2007;102:1307–11.

13. Ellrichmann M, Sergeev P, Bethge J, et al. Prospective evaluation of malignant cell seeding after percutaneous endoscopic gastrostomy in patients with oropharyngeal/esophageal cancers. Endoscopy 2013;45:526–31.

14. Vincenzi F, De Caro G, Gaiani F, et al. Risk of tumor implantation in percutaneous endoscopic gastrostomy in the upper aerodigestive tumors. Acta Biomed 2018; 89:117–21.

15. Kirby DF, Delegge MH, Fleming CR. American Gastroenterological Association technical review on tube feeding for enteral nutrition. Gastroenterology 1995; 108:1282–301.

16. Samarasena JB, Kwak NH, Chang KJ, et al. The PEG-Pedi-PEG technique: a novel method for percutaneous endoscopic gastrojejunostomy tube placement (with video). Gastrointest Endosc 2016;84:1030–3.

17. Dumot JA, Seidner DL. Direct button percutaneous endoscopic jejunostomy: successful placement in a patient with severe malnutrition and previous gastric resection. Gastrointest Endosc 1997;45:92–4.

18. Shike M, Latkany L. Direct percutaneous endoscopic jejunostomy. Gastrointest Endosc Clin N Am 1998;8:569–80.

19. Mackenzie SH, Haslem D, Hilden K, et al. Success rate of direct percutaneous endoscopic jejunostomy in patients who are obese. Gastrointest Endosc 2008; 67:265–9.

20. Deliwala SS, Chandan S, Kumar A, et al. Direct percutaneous endoscopic jejunostomy (DPEJ) and percutaneous endoscopic gastrostomy with jejunal extension (PEG-J) technical success and outcomes: Systematic review and meta-analysis. Endosc Int Open 2022;10:E488–520.

21. Gkolfakis P, Arvanitakis M, Despott EJ, et al. Endoscopic management of enteral tubes in adult patients - Part 2: Peri- and post-procedural management. European Society of Gastrointestinal Endoscopy (ESGE) Guideline. Endoscopy 2021;53:178–95.

22. Committee AT, Kwon RS, Banerjee S, et al. Enteral nutrition access devices. Gastrointest Endosc 2010;72:236–48.

23. Irani S, Kozarek RA. History of GI Stenting: Rigid Prostheses in the Esophagus. In: Kozarek R, Baron T, Song H-Y, editors. Self-expandable stents in the gastrointestinal tract. New York, NY: Springer New York; 2013. p. 3–13.

24. Sharma P, Kozarek R, Practice Parameters Committee of American College of G. Role of esophageal stents in benign and malignant diseases. Am J Gastroenterol 2010;105:258–73 [quiz: 274].

25. Burstow M, Kelly T, Panchani S, et al. Outcome of palliative esophageal stenting for malignant dysphagia: a retrospective analysis. Dis Esophagus 2009;22: 519–25.

26. Min YW, Jang EY, Jung JH, et al. Comparison between gastrostomy feeding and self-expandable metal stent insertion for patients with esophageal cancer and dysphagia. PLoS One 2017;12:e0179522.

27. Wang T, Wen Q, Zhang Y, et al. Percutaneous Gastrostomy Compared with Esophageal Stent Placement for the Treatment of Esophageal Cancer with Dysphagia. J Vasc Intervent Radiol 2021;32:1215–20.

28. Woo SM, Kim DH, Lee WJ, et al. Comparison of uncovered and covered stents for the treatment of malignant duodenal obstruction caused by pancreaticobiliary cancer. Surg Endosc 2013;27:2031–9.

29. Baron TH. Management of simultaneous biliary and duodenal obstruction: the endoscopic perspective. Gut Liver 2010;4(Suppl 1):S50–6.

30. ASoP Committee, Jue TL, Storm AC, et al. ASGE guideline on the role of endoscopy in the management of benign and malignant gastroduodenal obstruction. Gastrointest Endosc 2021;93:309–322 e4.

31. Khashab M, Alawad AS, Shin EJ, et al. Enteral stenting versus gastrojejunostomy for palliation of malignant gastric outlet obstruction. Surg Endosc 2013;27:2068–75.

32. Piesman M, Kozarek RA, Brandabur JJ, et al. Improved oral intake after palliative duodenal stenting for malignant obstruction: a prospective multicenter clinical trial. Am J Gastroenterol 2009;104:2404–11.

33. Song HY, Kim JH, Kim KR, et al. Malignant rectal obstruction within 5 cm of the anal verge: is there a role for expandable metallic stent placement? Gastrointest Endosc 2008;68:713–20.

34. Sebastian S, Johnston S, Geoghegan T, et al. Pooled analysis of the efficacy and safety of self-expanding metal stenting in malignant colorectal obstruction. Am J Gastroenterol 2004;99:2051–7.

35. van Halsema EE, van Hooft JE, Small AJ, et al. Perforation in colorectal stenting: a meta-analysis and a search for risk factors. Gastrointest Endosc 2014;79:970–82, e7; quiz 983 e2, 983 e5.

36. van Hooft JE, Veld JV, Arnold D, et al. Self-expandable metal stents for obstructing colonic and extracolonic cancer: European Society of Gastrointestinal Endoscopy (ESGE) Guideline - Update 2020. Endoscopy 2020;52:389–407.

37. Fritscher-Ravens A, Mosse CA, Mills TN, et al. A through-the-scope device for suturing and tissue approximation under EUS control. Gastrointest Endosc 2002;56: 737–42.

38. Binmoeller KF, Shah JN. Endoscopic ultrasound-guided gastroenterostomy using novel tools designed for transluminal therapy: a porcine study. Endoscopy 2012; 44:499–503.

39. Rimbaş M, Larghi A, Costamagna G. Endoscopic ultrasound-guided gastroenterostomy: Are we ready for prime time? Endoscopic Ultrasound 2017;6:235.

40. Khashab MA, Bukhari M, Baron TH, et al. International multicenter comparative trial of endoscopic ultrasonography-guided gastroenterostomy versus surgical gastrojejunostomy for the treatment of malignant gastric outlet obstruction. Endosc Int Open 2017;5:E275–81.

41. Itoi T, Ishii K, Ikeuchi N, et al. Prospective evaluation of endoscopic ultrasonography-guided double-balloon-occluded gastrojejunostomy bypass (EPASS) for malignant gastric outlet obstruction. Gut 2016;65:193–5.

42. Dzwonkowski M, Iqbal U, Berger A, et al. S1127 EUS-Guided Gastroenterostomy vs. Enteral Stenting for Palliation of Benign and Malignant Gastric Outlet Obstruction. Official journal of the American College of Gastroenterology| ACG 2022;117: e820–1.

43. Canakis A, Bomman S, Lee DU, et al. Benefits of EUS-Guided Gastroenterostomy Over Surgical Gastrojejunostomy in the Palliation of Malignant Gastric Outlet Obstruction: A Large Multicenter Experience. Gastrointest Endosc 2023. https://doi.org/10.1016/j.gie.2023.03.022.

Endoscopic Ultrasound-Guided Pain Management

Amirali Tavangar, MD, Jason B. Samarasena, MD, MBA*

KEYWORDS

- Pancreatic cancer • Endosonography • Celiac plexus neurolysis
- Celiac ganglia neurolysis • Endoscopic ultrasound

KEY POINTS

- Endoscopic ultrasound-guided celiac plexus neurolysis (EUS-CPN) is an alternative to chronic pain control with opiates in pancreatic cancer and chronic pancreatitis with the goal of improving quality of life.
- Due to the proximity of the celiac plexus to the GI tract, this approach is optimal for reaching the plexus and may be safer than a percutaneous approach.
- The goal of pain relief with EUS-guided celiac interventions is to help avoid chronic narcotic use or significantly reduce the dose to prevent narcotic addiction and its side effects.
- The volume of injectate may be an important consideration for the safety of this procedure, and injections greater than 20ml should generally be avoided.
- A novel approach has been EUS-guided radiofrequency ablation of the celiac ganglia by using a high-frequency alternating current to produce thermal coagulation of the ganglia tissue.

INTRODUCTION

Patients with pancreatic cancer (PC) are commonly diagnosed at an advanced stage and can be accompanied by severe abdominal pain for which management is often challenging. The pain etiology has been attributed to multiple causes such as increased intrapancreatic pressure, pancreatic ischemia, fibrosis, pseudocyst formation, and invasion of cancer cells to surrounding tissues.[1] Current pharmacologic management of pain involves starting with nonsteroidal anti-inflammatory drugs and then progressing to increasing doses of opioid analgesics.[2] However, opioids often provide suboptimal pain relief, and their use is limited by side effects such as constipation, urinary retention, nausea, confusion, somnolence, addiction, and developing

Division of Gastroenterology and Hepatology, Digestive Health Institute, University of California Irvine, Orange, CA, USA
* Corresponding author. Division of Gastroenterology and Hepatology, Suite 6400, 3800 West Chapman Avenue, Orange, CA 92868.
E-mail address: jsamaras@uci.edu

Gastrointest Endoscopy Clin N Am 34 (2024) 179–187
https://doi.org/10.1016/j.giec.2023.07.006
1052-5157/24/© 2023 Elsevier Inc. All rights reserved.
giendo.theclinics.com

tolerance.[3,4] The next step in pain management can be deactivation of the nociceptive neurons responsible for the pancreatic pain transmission by injection of local anesthetics (celiac block) or neurolytic agents such as absolute ethanol (celiac neurolysis). Given the shortened life expectancy of patients with PC, celiac neurolysis has been used in these patients with the goal of improving pain control and quality of life (QOL) while reducing the risk of drug-induced side effects. Traditionally, these procedures have been performed percutaneously, but the advent of linear endoscopic ultrasound (EUS) has given us the opportunity to do these interventions endoscopically through the gastric wall with several techniques. What follows is a detailed review of the technical aspects of the various procedural approaches and the current outcome evidence that exists.

RELEVANT ANATOMY

The celiac plexus is composed of a cluster of nerve cell bodies located just below the diaphragm anterior to the aorta, which surrounds the origin of the celiac trunk. Celiac ganglia might vary in number (usually 1–5), size (0.5 cm–4.5 cm), and location (T12–L2).[5] The celiac plexus is part of the autonomic nervous system, specifically the sympathetic division. They carry both sensory and motor fibers and can transmit pain sensation from the pancreas and most of the abdominal viscera except the left colon, rectum, and pelvic organs.[6]

PERCUTANEOUS CELIAC PLEXUS NEUROLYSIS

CPN can be performed through different routes percutaneously or under EUS guidance. Efficacy studies on percutaneous-guided celiac plexus neurolysis (PQ-CPN) for PC patients have shown mixed results but overall have demonstrated some benefit with fairly low risk. A Cochrane meta-analysis evaluated six randomized trials with 358 patients undergoing PQ-CPN for PC pain.[7] At 4 and 8 weeks, patients in the treatment arm had significant improvement in pain compared with the control arm. Furthermore, opioid consumption was significantly lower in the treatment arm. In another meta-analysis by Eisenberg and colleagues of 24 studies with 1145 patients treated with PQ-CPN for palliation of cancer pain (of which 63% were patients with PC), good to excellent pain relief was noted in 70% to 90% of patients up to 3 months after the procedure regardless of which type of percutaneous technique was used.[8]

A recent randomized controlled study by Yoon and colleagues compared the efficacy and safety of PQ-CPN and EUS-guided celiac plexus neurolysis (EUS-CPN).[9] Sixty PC patients with intractable pain were randomly assigned to EUS-CPN ($n = 30$) or PQ-CPN ($n = 30$). The two methods showed similar results in successful pain response, improvement of quality of life, patient satisfaction, incidence of adverse events, opioid requirement reduction, and survival rates at 3 months after intervention. They concluded that EUS-CPN and PQ-CPN were similarly effective and safe in managing intractable pain in PC patients and either methods may be used depending on the resources and expertise of each institution.

ENDOSCOPIC ULTRASOUND-GUIDED CELIAC PLEXUS NEUROLYSIS

EUS-CPN was originally described by Wiersema and colleagues[10] and involves diffuse injection into the region of the celiac plexus. This procedure is usually performed in the outpatient setting and sometimes during the index examination conducted for the purpose of PC diagnosis and staging. Contraindications to CPN in our practice include resectable PC, uncorrectable coagulopathy (international normalized ratio [INR] > 1.5), thrombocytopenia (platelets < 50,000/L), inadequate hydration, presence of esophageal or gastric varices, and altered anatomy prohibiting visualization or access to the celiac plexus/ganglia (such as gastric surgery or anomalies of the celiac trunk).[11] Patients are initially hydrated with 500 to 1000 mL of normal saline to minimize risk of hypotension. The procedure is performed with the patient in the left lateral decubitus position under moderate sedation or anesthesia. Continuous monitoring is necessary during and for 2 hours after the procedure. Before discharge, the blood pressure is rechecked in a supine and seated position to assess for orthostasis.[3] There is little evidence to support prophylactic antibiotics after CPN; thus, we do not routinely administer postprocedure antibiotics in our practice.

Endoscopic Ultrasound-Guided Celiac Plexus Neurolysis Efficacy

Within the literature, there is great variability among the studies in terms of injection technique, type of injectate and volume, and definition of pain relief and follow-up. For CPN, partial pain relief has been reported between 66% and 78% within the first 4 weeks.[12–15] In a randomized controlled trial (RCT), 96 patients with inoperable PC were randomized into conventional pain management or EUS-CPN. At 3 months, patients treated with CPN had greater pain relief with a trend toward lower morphine consumption, although no difference was observed in quality of life.[16] Overall, three meta-analyses have reported approximately 53% to 73% pain reduction for 2 to 4 weeks with EUS-CPN.[17–19]

Of note, a recent RCT by Kanno and colleagues on 48 unresectable PC patients showed no benefit of EUS-CPN over medical therapy with oxycodone/fentanyl.[20] EUS-CPN was successfully performed and did not induce severe procedure-related adverse events for all patients in the EUS-CPN group. Although the average pain scores for both groups significantly decreased in comparison with baseline, scores were not statistically different between the groups at week 4. There was no statistical difference or tendency in favor of EUS-CPN at evaluation points of weeks 1, 2, 8, and 12. Moreover, the average scores for QOL and the average opioid consumption between the groups were not different at all evaluation points.

Endoscopic Ultrasound-Guided Celiac Plexus Neurolysis Technique

Celiac plexus injection was the first described and is currently the most widely performed technique.[10] Linear array endosonographic imaging from the proximal posterior stomach allows visualization of the aorta, which seems in a longitudinal plane. The aorta is traced distally to the celiac trunk, which is the first major branch below the diaphragm. Targeting with CPN is based on the expected location of the celiac plexus relative to the celiac trunk and Doppler should be used to clearly delineate vascular structures. In our practice, a standard 22-gauge needle without stylet is primed with the injectant and inserted through the scope working channel and affixed at the inlet. The needle is then advanced under EUS guidance until the needle tip is placed approximately 5 to 10 mm away from the origin of the celiac trunk. Either the entire injectate volume is inserted in the midline position (central approach) or half of the injectate is inserted onto each side of the celiac takeoff (bilateral approach). An aspiration test is performed to rule out vascular penetration before each injection.[21]

Neurolytic agent

Although the types and volumes of injectate differ, for patients with PC, we typically inject a premixed 10 mL solution of 98% ethanol alcohol and 0.75% bupivacaine in a 70:30 ratio. As an alternative in patients with alcohol intolerance (aldehyde dehydrogenase deficiency), Ishiwatari and colleagues investigated the use of phenol as compared with ethanol as their neurolytic agent and found no differences in pain control or complications.[22]

Volume of injectate

The volume of alcohol used in EUS-CPN has not been standardized, and the reports have ranged between 10 and as high as 23 mL.[23] Leblanc and colleagues conducted a prospective pilot study comparing the safety of 20 mL versus 10 mL of alcohol during EUS-CPN. There was no difference in pain relief, duration of pain relief, and adverse events between the two groups. They concluded that using 20 mL of alcohol is safe.[24] Of note, there was a report of a serious complication by Fuji and colleagues following CPN where a patient had an anterior spinal cord infarction resulting in permanent paralysis. In this report, the patient underwent injection with 23 mL of alcohol.[23] It is difficult to know if the higher volume played a major role in this complication, but in our practice, we rarely exceed 15 mL of injectate.

Unilateral versus bilateral

In the bilateral technique, we inject half the volume on the left side of the celiac origin and the remainder at the mid-line at the takeoff. Our rationale for this modified technique is that the right side of the celiac artery is not as accessible, given the slight tilt of the artery relative to the scope position. Therefore, left and mid-line are the preferred areas for injection. However, some prefer to inject at a single site, usually midline (central approach).

A meta-analysis by Lu and colleagues of 437 patients with six studies, including three RCTs, compared bilateral and unilateral CPN for PC.[25] Despite there being no significant difference in short-term pain relief between the two groups, the bilateral approach was associated with a statistically significant reduction in analgesic use compared with the unilateral approach. In contrast, a prior meta-analysis found that a significantly higher proportion of patients with bilateral injection had higher rates of pain relief compared with unilateral injection (84.5% vs 46%).[26] A clinical practice guideline from 2017 on EUS-CPN has suggested the use of bilateral injection, but also states that a central injection is acceptable.[27]

ENDOSCOPIC ULTRASOUND-GUIDED BROAD PLEXUS NEUROLYSIS

An alternative approach, first described by Sakamoto and colleagues which may be more applicable to advanced abdominal cancer patients, is EUS-guided broad plexus neurolysis (BPN). In this study, a 25-gauge needle was used to perform an injection at the level of the superior mesenteric artery resulting in a broader distribution of neurolysis. BPN had significantly better 7-day and 30-day pain relief scores as compared with conventional EUS-CPN.[28] Since this original study, there has yet to be further studies comparing BPN versus conventional EUS-CPN.

Endoscopic Ultrasound-Guided Direct Celiac Ganglion Neurolysis

Recently, it has been recognized that the individual celiac ganglia can be visualized and accessed by EUS allowing for direct injection into the individual celiac ganglia to perform celiac ganglion neurolysis (CGN). The celiac ganglia are typically oval or almond-shaped ranging in size between 2 and 20 mm and most readily detected to the left of the celiac artery, anterior to the aorta. Compared with the surrounding retroperitoneal fat, the ganglia are echo poor and often display similar echogenicity to the left adrenal gland. Within the ganglia, often central echo-rich strands and foci are present and the margins of the ganglia are irregular. Color Doppler demonstrates little to

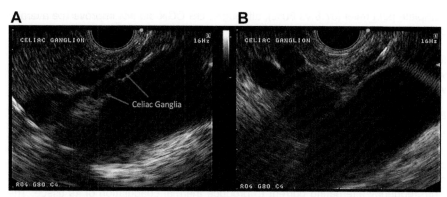

Fig. 1. EUS-guided direct injection of alcohol into two celiac ganglia in a patient with pancreatic cancer. (*A*) Linear EUS view identifying celiac ganglia. (*B*) Linear EUS view with celiac ganglion being injected and ballooning demonstrated.

no flow within these structures. Ganglia are detected by EUS in between 81% and 89% of patients.[29]

All aspects of the procedure including patient candidacy, sedation, antibiotic use, and follow-up are the same as standard CPN. The technique for CGN and volume of solution injected has not been standardized. Our approach is to target as many ganglia as possible by injecting a total of 10 to 20 mL of premixed alcohol and bupivacaine (mixture as outlined earlier) among all the ganglia in amounts relative to their size. For example, if there are three ganglia visualized, small-, medium-, and large-sized, we would typically inject 5 mL in the largest ganglion, 3 mL in the medium-sized ganglion, and 2 mL in the small ganglion. For larger ganglia, we typically advance the needle tip into the deepest point within the ganglia, and then inject while slowly withdrawing the needle creating an even distribution of injectate throughout the ganglion. For smaller ganglia, we usually target the ganglia's center. During injection, a clear "ballooning" of the ganglia should be visualized otherwise needle placement is considered suboptimal (**Fig. 1**).

In a prospective trial by Doi and colleagues comparing CGN to CPN, 68 patients with upper abdominal cancer (85% PC) were randomly assigned to treatment using either EUS-CGN or EUS-CPN with one midline injection. The positive response rate was significantly higher in the EUS-CGN group (73.5%) than in the EUS-CPN group (45.5%). The complete response rate, defined as greater than 50% reduction at 12 weeks, was also significantly higher in the EUS-CGN group (50%) than in the EUS-CPN group (18.2%). There was no difference in adverse events or duration of pain relief between the groups.[30] Follow-up was only 7 days and there were no patients included with bilateral EUS-CPN injections. A randomized double-blinded prospective study of 110 patients by Levy and colleagues with unresectable PC showed that patients who underwent combined CGN + CPN actually had a shorter median survival time compared with patients who underwent CPN alone (5.6 vs 10.5 months), but no significant difference in pain control, quality of life, and opioid intake. This study raised concerns about the appropriateness of CGN in combination with CGN for patients with PC.[31]

In a more recent prospective study by Kamata and colleagues, 51 consecutive patients with PC-associated pain where enrolled in EUS-CPN and then EUS-CGN were added in cases of visible celiac ganglia. Ganglia were visible in 41 patients and results showed that EUS-CPN plus EUS-CGN was superior to EUS-CPN alone for achieving complete pain relief (87.8 vs 60%), although EUS-CGN did not improve the average duration of the pain relief.[32]

A recent qualitative systematic review by Li and colleagues involving 319 patients found that EUS-CGN seemed to correlate with better pain response at 1 week, whereas long-term results showed a great deal of variability and it may shorten survival compared with patients undergoing EUS-CPN.[33]

Endoscopic Ultrasound-Guided Radiofrequency Ablation of Celiac Ganglia

A novel approach to PC pain control has been EUS-guided radiofrequency ablation (RFA) of the celiac ganglia, being first reported by Jin and colleagues in a single case report. This is a procedure by which ganglia are destroyed using a thin needle-like electrode, which is inserted into the target ganglion and then ablated using high-frequency alternating current to produce thermal coagulation of its tissue. The original technique by Jin and colleagues involved using the Habib monopolar RFA probe (EMcision Ltd, London, UK), which was inserted inside the hollow of a 19-gauge fine needle aspiration (FNA) needle after removal of the stylet until the needle tip is reached. The ganglia were then punctured and the needle was then withdrawn slightly as the RFA catheter was simultaneously advanced. Ablation was done until the center of the ganglion gradually became hyperechoic on EUS. The investigators were able to show significant improvement in patient's pain as well as eliminating the need for further opiate medication.[34]

A recent randomized trial of RFA versus fine needle ethanol injection was performed by Bang and colleagues on 26 patients with 14 cases undergoing EUS-CPN and 12 cases of EUS-RFA. Pain severity, quality of life, and opioid use were compared among the groups. This trial suggested clinical superiority of RFA, demonstrated by significantly more improvement in pain scores, fewer postprocedural gastrointestinal symptoms, and better emotional functioning compared with the EUS-CPN group. Importantly, they showed 21% of patients with persistent pain after CPN could be successfully managed with RFA.[35]

In another study by Houmani and colleagues, a novel RFA EUS needle (Starmed, Taewoong Medical, Seoul, South Korea) was used in two patients and showed significant pain reduction without any adverse events.[36]

This seems to be a promising approach for two reasons; first, EUS-CPN effect is often short-lived and despite its frequent use and data supporting its effectiveness, it has been associated with a significant variation in analgesic effectiveness for patients with PC pain (24%–80%).[37] In comparison, RFA induces irreparable cellular damage and coagulation necrosis of the ganglion tissue; therefore, it might afford patients more long-lasting pain relief. Second, EUS-RFA can allow stricter control of the ablated zone and a more predictable area of necrosis and therefore can produce immediate pain relief and less collateral damage than alcohol injection.[38,39] However, some doubt the cost-effectives of this approach given RFA probes are much more expensive than the cost of alcohol.[40] Overall, the data on EUS-RFA are limited but promising; further studies are needed to further refine this technique and show long-term durability and prove cost-effectiveness.

COMPLICATIONS

Most complications related to CPN and CGN are transient, and serious complications are rare. The most common side effects reported are transient hypotension (up to 35%), diarrhea (up to 20%), and transient exacerbation of pain following procedure, which are consistent with rates seen with the percutaneous approach.[8] Hypotension and diarrhea are related to sympathetic blockade and the relative unopposed visceral parasympathetic activity. Hypotension generally responds to intravenous (IV) fluid administration. The diarrhea related to this procedure is usually self-limiting and resolves in less than 48 hours. CPN via a percutaneous approach has been associated with a 2% rate of serious complications including neurologic complications (lower extremity weakness, paresthesia, paralysis), pain (pleuritic chest, shoulder), pneumothorax, and hiccupping.[8] A very small number of serious complications ($\leq$0.6%) including fatalities and paralysis mainly with alcohol injection have been reported with the EUS approach in case report and abstract form.[23,41,42]

SUMMARY

Performing EUS-guided CPN and CGN has been a mainstay for the endoscopic oncologist managing patients with PC. Studies clearly demonstrate that CPN and CGN aid in reducing pain that is refractory to medical therapy. There remains to be a great deal of practice variability with regard to the injectate volume, type, and optimal location of the injection. However, more recent randomized data are starting to shape best practice. The advent of CGN using RFA likely marks the next phase in the evolution of EUS-guided pain control for patients with PC, and we look forward to more studies using this ablative modality and others.

CLINICS CARE POINTS

- Patient selection is key to finding the patient who can benefit most from this procedure.
- EUS guided approach to celiac plexus/ganglion interventions is safe.
- When the response to the treatment is not complete, repeating the procedure could result in an additional response.

REFERENCES

1. Yan BM, Myers RP. Neurolytic celiac plexus block for pain control in unresectable pancreatic cancer. Am J Gastroenterol 2007;102(2):430–8.
2. Ventafridda V, Tamburini M, Caraceni A, et al. A validation study of the WHO method for cancer pain relief. Cancer 1987;59(4):850–6.
3. Levy MJ, Chari ST, Wiersema MJ. Endoscopic ultrasound-guided celiac neurolysis. Gastrointest Endosc Clin N Am 2012;22(2):231–47, viii.
4. Yeager MP, Colacchio TA, Yu CT, et al. Morphine inhibits spontaneous and cytokine-enhanced natural killer cell cytotoxicity in volunteers. Anesthesiology 1995;83(3):500–8.
5. Ward EM, Rorie DK, Nauss LA, et al. The celiac ganglia in man: normal anatomic variations. Anesth Analg 1979;58(6):461–5.
6. Brown DL, Moore DC. The use of neurolytic celiac plexus block for pancreatic cancer: anatomy and technique. J Pain Symptom Manage 1988;3(4):206–9.
7. Arcidiacono PG, Calori G, Carrara S, et al. Celiac plexus block for pancreatic cancer pain in adults. Cochrane Database Syst Rev 2011;2011(3):CD007519.
8. Eisenberg E, Carr DB, Chalmers TC. Neurolytic celiac plexus block for treatment of cancer pain: a meta-analysis. Anesth Analg 1995;80(2):290–5.

9. Yoon WJ, Oh Y, Yoo C, et al. EUS-Guided Versus Percutaneous Celiac Neurolysis for the Management of Intractable Pain Due to Unresectable Pancreatic Cancer: A Randomized Clinical Trial. J Clin Med 2020;9(6).

10. Wiersema MJ, Wiersema LM. Endosonography-guided celiac plexus neurolysis. Gastrointest Endosc 1996;44(6):656–62.

11. Pérez-Aguado G, de la Mata DM, Valenciano CM, Sainz IF. Endoscopic ultrasonography-guided celiac plexus neurolysis in patients with unresectable pancreatic cancer: An update. World J Gastrointest Endosc 2021;13(10):460–72.

12. Gunaratnam NT, Sarma AV, Norton ID, et al. A prospective study of EUS-guided celiac plexus neurolysis for pancreatic cancer pain. Gastrointest Endosc 2001; 54(3):316–24.

13. Iwata K, Yasuda I, Enya M, et al. Predictive factors for pain relief after endoscopic ultrasound-guided celiac plexus neurolysis. Dig Endosc 2011;23(2):140–5.

14. Seicean A, Cainap C, Gulei I, et al. Pain palliation by endoscopic ultrasound-guided celiac plexus neurolysis in patients with unresectable pancreatic cancer. J Gastrointestin Liver Dis 2013;22(1):59–64.

15. Sahai AV, Lemelin V, Lam E, et al. Central vs. bilateral endoscopic ultrasound-guided celiac plexus block or neurolysis: a comparative study of short-term effectiveness. Am J Gastroenterol 2009;104(2):326–9.

16. Wyse JM, Carone M, Paquin SC, et al. Randomized, double-blind, controlled trial of early endoscopic ultrasound-guided celiac plexus neurolysis to prevent pain progression in patients with newly diagnosed, painful, inoperable pancreatic cancer. J Clin Oncol 2011;29(26):3541–6.

17. Koulouris AI, Alexandre L, Hart AR, Clark A. Endoscopic ultrasound-guided celiac plexus neurolysis (EUS-CPN) technique and analgesic efficacy in patients with pancreatic cancer: A systematic review and meta-analysis. Pancreatology 2021;21(2):434–42.

18. Kaufman M, Singh G, Das S, et al. Efficacy of endoscopic ultrasound-guided celiac plexus block and celiac plexus neurolysis for managing abdominal pain associated with chronic pancreatitis and pancreatic cancer. J Clin Gastroenterol 2010;44(2):127–34.

19. Asif AA, Walayat SK, Bechtold ML, et al. EUS-guided celiac plexus neurolysis for pain in pancreatic cancer patients - a meta-analysis and systematic review. J Community Hosp Intern Med Perspect 2021;11(4):536–42.

20. Kanno Y, Koshita S, Masu K, et al. Efficacy of EUS-guided celiac plexus neurolysis compared with medication alone for unresectable pancreatic cancer in the oxycodone/fentanyl era: a prospective randomized control study. Gastrointest Endosc 2020;92(1):120–30.

21. Fujii-Lau LL, Wiersema MJ, Levy MJ. Celiac Plexus Blockade/Neurolysis. In: Facciorusso A, Muscatiello N, editors. Endoscopic ultrasound management of pancreatic Lesions: from diagnosis to therapy. Cham: Springer International Publishing; 2021. p. 201–10.

22. Ishiwatari H, Hayashi T, Yoshida M, et al. Phenol-based endoscopic ultrasound-guided celiac plexus neurolysis for East Asian alcohol-intolerant upper gastrointestinal cancer patients: a pilot study. World J Gastroenterol: WJG 2014;20(30):10512.

23. Fujii L, Clain JE, Morris JM, Levy MJ. Anterior spinal cord infarction with permanent paralysis following endoscopic ultrasound celiac plexus neurolysis. Endoscopy. 2012;44 Suppl 2 UCTN:E265-6. doi: 10.1055/s-0032-1309708.

24. Leblanc JK, Rawl S, Juan M, et al. Endoscopic Ultrasound-Guided Celiac Plexus Neurolysis in Pancreatic Cancer: A Prospective Pilot Study of Safety Using 10 mL versus 20 mL Alcohol. Diagn Ther Endosc 2013;2013:327036.

25. Lu F, Dong J, Tang Y, et al. Bilateral vs. unilateral endoscopic ultrasound-guided celiac plexus neurolysis for abdominal pain management in patients with pancreatic malignancy: a systematic review and meta-analysis. Support Care Cancer 2018;26(2):353–9.

26. Puli SR, Reddy JB, Bechtold ML, et al. EUS-guided celiac plexus neurolysis for pain due to chronic pancreatitis or pancreatic cancer pain: a meta-analysis and systematic review. Dig Dis Sci 2009;54(11):2330–7.

27. Wyse JM, Battat R, Sun S, et al. Practice guidelines for endoscopic ultrasound-guided celiac plexus neurolysis. Endosc Ultrasound 2017;6(6):369–75.

28. Sakamoto H, Kitano M, Kamata K, et al. EUS-guided broad plexus neurolysis over the superior mesenteric artery using a 25-gauge needle. Am J Gastroenterol 2010;105(12):2599–606.

29. Gleeson FC, Levy MJ, Papachristou GI, et al. Frequency of visualization of presumed celiac ganglia by endoscopic ultrasound. Endoscopy 2007;39(7):620–4.

30. Doi S, Yasuda I, Kawakami H, et al. Endoscopic ultrasound-guided celiac ganglia neurolysis vs. celiac plexus neurolysis: a randomized multicenter trial. Endoscopy 2013;45(5):362–9.

31. Levy MJ, Gleeson FC, Topazian MD, et al. Combined Celiac Ganglia and Plexus Neurolysis Shortens Survival, Without Benefit, vs Plexus Neurolysis Alone. Clin Gastroenterol Hepatol 2019;17(4):728–38.e9.

32. Kamata K, Kinoshita M, Kinoshita I, et al. Efficacy of EUS-guided celiac plexus neurolysis in combination with EUS-guided celiac ganglia neurolysis for pancreatic cancer-associated pain: a multicenter prospective trial. Int J Clin Oncol 2022; 27(7):1196–201.

33. Li M, Wang Z, Chen Y, et al. EUS-CGN versus EUS-CPN in pancreatic cancer: A qualitative systematic review. Medicine (Baltimore) 2021;100(41):e27103.

34. Jin ZD, Wang L, Li Z. Endoscopic ultrasound-guided celiac ganglion radiofrequency ablation for pain control in pancreatic carcinoma. Dig Endosc 2015; 1(27):163–4.

35. Bang JY, Sutton B, Hawes RH, Varadarajulu S. EUS-guided celiac ganglion radiofrequency ablation versus celiac plexus neurolysis for palliation of pain in pancreatic cancer: a randomized controlled trial (with videos). Gastrointest Endosc 2019;89(1):58–66.e3.

36. Houmani ZS, Noureddine MS. EUS-guided celiac plexus radiofrequency ablation using a novel device. VideoGIE 2020;5(9):395–6.

37. Benson M, Pfau P. Pain relief and the celiac plexus: Can burning exceed injecting? Gastrointest Endosc 2019;89(1):67–8.

38. Vanella G, Capurso G, Arcidiacono PG. Endosonography-guided Radiofrequency Ablation in Pancreatic Diseases: Time to Fill the Gap Between Evidence and Enthusiasm. J Clin Gastroenterol 2020;54(7):591–601.

39. Moutinho-Ribeiro P, Costa-Moreira P, Caldeira A, et al. Endoscopic Ultrasound-Guided Celiac Plexus Interventions. GE Port J Gastroenterol 2020;28(1):32–8.

40. Larghi A, Rimbaş M, Crinò SF. EUS-guided radiofrequency ablation of the celiac axis in pancreatic cancer: Is money worth the pain? Gastrointest Endosc 2019; 89(1):207.

41. Alvarez-Sanchez MV, Jenssen C, Faiss S, et al. Interventional endoscopic ultrasonography: an overview of safety and complications. Surg Endosc 2014;28(3): 712–34.

42. Loeve US, Mortensen MB. Lethal necrosis and perforation of the stomach and the aorta after multiple EUS-guided celiac plexus neurolysis procedures in a patient with chronic pancreatitis. Gastrointest Endosc 2013;77(1):151–2.

Moving?

Make sure your subscription moves with you!

To notify us of your new address, find your **Clinics Account Number** (located on your mailing label above your name), and contact customer service at:

Email: journalscustomerservice-usa@elsevier.com

800-654-2452 (subscribers in the U.S. & Canada)
314-447-8871 (subscribers outside of the U.S. & Canada)

Fax number: 314-447-8029

Elsevier Health Sciences Division
Subscription Customer Service
3251 Riverport Lane
Maryland Heights, MO 63043

*To ensure uninterrupted delivery of your subscription, please notify us at least 4 weeks in advance of move.

Printed and bound by CPI Group (UK) Ltd, Croydon, CR0 4YY

08/05/2025

01864750-0009